"This is a fantastic, accessible introduction to visual perception [...] eyes-on approach to teaching perception will help students eng[...] stand the content."

Dr. Julia Stra

"Ben Balas' book gives a much-needed new perspective on what a Sensation & Perception course can and should do for students. Vision research is all about how we see the world, and Balas' book provides carefully structured exercises that encourage students to see and understand for themselves how their vision works. With its hands-on experiments and accompanying text, Balas' approach all but guarantees that what students learn will not soon be forgotten (something all teachers can only aspire to)."

Dr. Robert Sekuler, *Brandeis University, USA*

"This is a wonderfully original textbook, quite unlike anything else on the market. It's packed with brilliant hands-on exercises to inspire students and teachers alike. Prof. Balas leads the reader step-by-step to a deep understanding of how and why the visual system works the way it does through compelling demos that you can try out for yourself at home, in the lab or in the lecture hall."

Dr. Roland Fleming, *University of Giessen,*
Germany

Practical Vision Science

This workbook provides a collection of experiments and observations that use physical materials (rather than digital displays or resources) to reveal fundamental properties of the human visual system.

Practical Vision Science centers discovery, observation, and critical thinking. By observing and manipulating visual phenomena, readers gain insights regarding visual processing from the outside world into high-level areas of the visual cortex. The text covers geometric optics, image formation, early stages of visual processing, and inferences regarding brightness, color, depth, motion, and form. The goal is to highlight the critical role that observation of one's own sensory experiences plays in vision science, while introducing phenomena that provide clues about the computations and constraints that shape our experience of the visual world. Each exercise can be completed with everyday materials, and the text includes discussion of key phenomena readers should be able to observe and the implications of these effects for underlying mechanisms that support visual experience in each case.

Practical Vision Science is an essential text for upper undergraduate and postgraduate students of Sensation and Perception, providing the opportunity to learn by doing things rather than reading facts about the visual system on the page.

Benjamin Balas is a Professor of Psychology at North Dakota State University, USA. He received both his SB and PhD from MIT's Department of Brain and Cognitive Sciences and completed post-doctoral work at Children's Hospital Boston.

Practical Vision Science
Learning Through Experimentation

Benjamin Balas

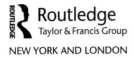

NEW YORK AND LONDON

Designed cover image: Jolygon via Getty Images

First published 2025

by Routledge
605 Third Avenue, New York, NY 10158

and by Routledge
4 Park Square, Milton Park, Abingdon, Oxon, OX14 4RN

Routledge is an imprint of the Taylor & Francis Group, an informa business

© 2025 Benjamin Balas

ISBN: 978-1-032-69115-2 (hbk)
ISBN: 978-1-032-69112-1 (pbk)
ISBN: 978-1-032-69116-9 (ebk)

DOI: 10.4324/9781032691169

Typeset in Galliard
by Deanta Global Publishing Services, Chennai, India

Access the Support Material: www.routledge.com/9781032691121

To my daughter, Blaise, who has always kept a sharp eye out for what's interesting.

Contents

Acknowledgments   *x*

Introduction   1

1   What Is Light and What Does It Do?   5

2   Image Formation in the Eye   26

3   Measuring Light with the Retina   44

4   Spatial Vision in the LGN and V1   61

5   Perceptual Organization and Gestalt Principles   78

6   Brightness and Color Constancy   90

7   Depth Perception   103

8   Motion Perception   126

9   Face Perception   138

Index   *147*

Acknowledgments

This is a modest book, but I hope it conveys how much I love vision science. I owe that love of seeing and thinking about what I see to a number of people that I would like to thank here.

Ted Adelson and Bart Anderson were the instructors for my first vision class, and I also count myself fortunate that Roland Fleming was my TA. The three of them each conveyed how much they loved vision science and clearly hoped we would love it too. In particular, I still remember the day that Bart told us he was worried we were getting too bogged down in words and equations, so he brought a turntable, some lights, and a bunch of other neat stuff to show us his favorite visual phenomena for an hour or so. That class session may be as close as I can get to pinpointing the exact moment that I knew I wanted to be a vision scientist myself. Thanks to all three of them for showing me how much fun vision could be.

While I'm not the most avid user of social media, I've been grateful for the community of vision scientists on various platforms who routinely share interesting and surprising visual effects, insights about vision from their own research, and ideas for teaching vision science at the university level. I will likely forget someone in this list, but many thanks to Gavin Buckingham, Steve Dakin, Will Harrison, Akiyoshi Kitaoka, Steve Most, Richard Prather, Ruth Rosenholtz, Bob Sekuler, Julia Strand, Sam Strong, Tim Vickery, Ben Wolfe, and Brad Wyble for being inspiring and fun people to share ideas with.

Finally, there are a few more people who deserve special praise. My wife and colleague, Erin Conwell, has encouraged me to try to be a better teacher through her own example and to commit to the ideas for my class that I'm most passionate about. For her support, her humor, and her insights about how (and why) to teach, I am ever grateful. My colleagues in the Psychology Department at NDSU have also been supportive of my efforts to transform our S&P (Sensation and Perception) class into something more interactive, and I'm thankful to work at an institution that has given me the freedom to teach my class in a way that makes it my own. Thanks especially to Jeff Johnson, Mark McCourt, and Laura Thomas for their support of my work in the classroom and their suggestions for other ways to make all of our classes engaging and informative. Also, I owe Lisa Scott a great debt for telling me, "You should write a textbook," at VSS Demo Night in 2023. Sometimes hearing a friend say it is the final push you need to believe something is actually a good idea.

Last, but not least, thanks to the students in my Psyc460 classes who have gamely built paper models, squinted at stereograms, held sunprint paper up to the sky on blisteringly cold (but clear!) winter days in Fargo, and stuck with me as I've developed and refined the exercises presented here. I hope you all learned something about vision, and I hope you had some fun doing so.

Introduction

What you have in front of you is a workbook designed to provide you with an introduction to vision science. This particular workbook is a collection of exercises using analog materials that I've developed for use in my upper division Sensation and Perception class at North Dakota State University in Fargo, ND ("North of Normal" – I wish I were kidding, but that really is our city's motto). There are of course many other textbooks that provide coverage of this material, so you'd be forgiven for asking "Why another one?" or "Why *this* one?" My hope is to use the first few pages of this book to answer these questions and both convince you that this workbook offers something interesting and unique and give you some pointers regarding how best to engage with it.

In many textbooks, I think we make a crucial mistake: We present our discipline (whether it's vision science or anything else) as a *fait accompli* without giving students much of an idea of how we arrived at the theories and models that offer our best understanding of the topic. On one hand, it's fair to spare students the messiness of having to reinvent the wheel – we all stand on the shoulders of giants, after all. On the other hand, I think that getting access to information about how we learned the things that we know can often make it easier to keep complicated concepts in mind. Perhaps more importantly, I think teaching science this way does a lot to communicate to students that scientific discovery is a process that they can take part in.

In many disciplines, it's a challenge to present introductory material this way without a lot of supporting infrastructure like lab space, chemicals, temperature-controlled equipment, and who knows what else. In vision science, by comparison, I think we have both an incredible opportunity to build instruction around discovery and few excuses not to do so. I say this because, compared to other fields, the basic data that we are trying to understand in vision science is immediately accessible for essentially no cost. Open your eyes, look around at the world, and there you have it: What can you see? Why do things look the way that they look? What successes and what mistakes do you make with your visual sense? At its core, vision science is built on this act of looking at the world and thinking about why it looks that way, both of which are not so difficult to do in a lab, a classroom, or the comfort of your own home.

I am of course not the first person to make this observation about vision science and link it to instruction. Demonstrations of visual phenomena play a huge role in the classroom already, and every one of my colleagues does *something* during the course of a Sensation and Perception class to show off a compelling illusion, an interesting quirk of the visual system, or to demonstrate the impressive capabilities of human vision. My own love of vision science came from watching my instructors struggle to make the Gelb staircase demo work with an overhead projector and a clothesline or use a record player to show off

DOI: 10.4324/9781032691169-1

different structure-from-motion patterns. Here's the thing, though: While demonstrations like this are fairly common in the classroom, I think most instructors (myself included for a long time) think of them more like interesting ornaments to add to a lecture instead of something fundamental to learning. The goal of this workbook is to center these activities so that students learn key concepts in vision science by starting with observation as much as possible, then linking observation to the theories and models that help account for what they saw. Broadly speaking, this is in keeping with the academic literature that supports active learning rather than more traditional, passive approaches. If I may be less formal for a moment, it's also a lot more fun.

Here is one important feature of the book that we should discuss, however. These days there are many excellent digital resources available online to show different visual phenomena, many of which make it possible to play with stimulus variables that are just not practical to manipulate without a monitor, tablet, or other fancy display. I use a lot of these resources too, but I have a special place in my heart for demonstrations that rely on physical stuff that you can hold, fiddle with, and observe right in front of you. Besides the fact that I may just be a bit of a Luddite who likes avoiding technology when I can, I think these kinds of analog demonstrations do a lot to convince students that there really are interesting visual phenomena to see and think about. Digital displays can deliver beautiful and vivid visual experiences, but I think that they also admit the possibility that what we're seeing may be more like a special effect than a real phenomenon. I'm not sure if that's actually an issue for the students I have worked with in the classroom, but I can tell you that seeing visual effects play out on your desk using lasers, holes punched in paper, and other ordinary materials carries just a little bit of magic. For that reason, I have structured the book around demonstrations and exercises that can be carried out using real materials, which in most cases are fairly inexpensive. This takes additional work and a little more time, but I think it's well worth it.

To say a bit about implementing this approach, if you intend to work your way through the whole textbook, there will be a need to invest in some *stuff*. The students in my class purchase a course kit – pictured in Figure 0.1 – containing most of the items needed to complete the exercises described in each chapter. There are a few exceptions (e.g. special light sources like strobes or UV lights), but these are relatively few and far between. I've listed the materials you need for each exercise, but I've avoided naming specific vendors because these are bound to become outdated sooner or later. Most everything here is available at fairly low cost, though, especially if you're able to purchase things in bulk. Also, many of the exercises described here can be accomplished using print-outs and ordinary office supplies (Figure 0.1).

Speaking of print-outs, you'll see that there are a number of exercises that make use of pictures or patterns that I've included as supplementary materials available for download from the publisher. In a few cases, there may be some benefit in trying to print these out on cardstock or another stiffer material, but this is not necessary: You can make everything work with ordinary printer paper. I do recommend investing in a good Exacto blade and a hole punch, however – cheap scissors will be the end of you by the end of a semester-long course if you're not careful.

With all that in mind, the overall plan I have for you in this book is to make structured observations of different visual phenomena, each one providing insight into some aspect of how the visual system works. The text is organized as a tour of the visual system from the outside world inward, beginning with the physics of light, image formation in the eye, and sensory transduction in the retina, then onward to pattern vision, color perception, motion

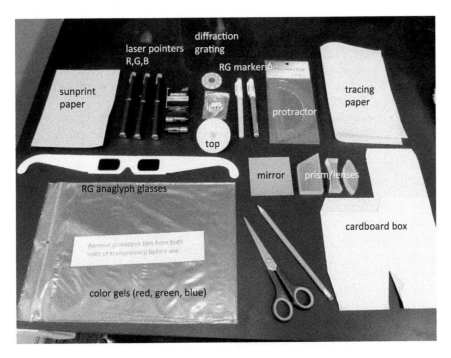

Figure 0.1 The course kit students in my Sensation and Perception class receive to complete the exercises described in the text. Photo by the author.

and depth perception, and face recognition. Accompanying each exercise, I've included some explication of what each set of effects tells us about the visual system, whether that's a clue to the underlying anatomy, hints of what the computational processes are that support our visual abilities, or connections between different sections of the workbook. This is where I need to give you some caveats, however, because while this may seem like a lot of material (and easily supports my semester-long course in Sensation and Perception) there are also a number of topics that I do not cover in this text. I think these exclusions are not so terrible, but if this is material you want to cover you will need to find some supporting resources to do so.

- My treatment of the anatomy of the visual system is relatively sparse as is my description of specific computations. There are many more details one could cover with regard to the cells in the retina, striate and extrastriate cortex, etc., and one could also expand on the quantitative models that account for the phenomena described here. At present, I've chosen to primarily offer pointers towards key computational ideas, using anatomy and physiology to reinforce key ideas in these areas. For an advanced treatment of the computational principles introduced here, John Frisby and James Stone's *Seeing* (2010) is an excellent resource.
- The book also does not cover psychophysical methods at all. My thinking here is that these reflect formal methods of measuring visual abilities in tightly controlled environments, and the perspective I am trying to offer in this text is one grounded in everyday visual experience. These are interesting and important ideas for students to know about,

however, and there are excellent resources for giving students short psychophysical experiments to carry out and analyze available from many places online. In the interests of highlighting analog demonstrations as much as possible, I have to mention the "Fech Deck" developed by Dr. James Ferwerda at the Rochester Institute of Technology (Ferwerda, 2019), which makes psychophysical testing possible with a deck of customized playing cards. Also, Palmer & Palmer's *Vision Science* (1999) is a classic text that covers psychophysical approaches in detail.

- The text also does not highlight individual vision scientists in a historical context or make many connections to specific people who contributed to the development of these ideas. This is also deliberate and motivated by my hope that by positioning students as investigators via a practical approach, we may make it easier for them to understand the nature of scientific inquiry and how they can participate in it. My feeling is that hearing a great deal about various "great names" in the field may make it less evident to students that vision science remains an exciting field with open questions that they could contribute to solving.

- You also will not find discussion here regarding the debates between various theoretical camps in the discipline. Again, the idea is to focus on what is discoverable and interpretable about day-to-day visual experience, and some of these theoretical perspectives require a more abstract synthesis of the field that I have found beyond the scope of what I'm trying to do in an introductory course.

So: That is what is here, what isn't here, and why you'll find what you find in the text. Please have fun playing with the lasers, mirrors, lenses, pinholes, tops, patterns, and pictures described here. Doing so will show you a lot of the interesting and at times puzzling work that your visual system is engaged in all the time. You can learn a lot by looking, and I hope this workbook gets you started down that path.

References

Ferwerda, J. (2019). The FechDeck: A hand tool for exploring psychophysics. *Transactions on Applied Perception, 16*, 1–14.

Frisby, J., & Stone, J. V. (2010). *Seeing: The computational approach to biological vision.* MIT Press.

Palmer, S. E., & Palmer, L. A. (1999). *Vision science: From photon to phenomenology.* MIT Press.

1 What Is Light and What Does It Do?

Before we can talk about how your visual system processes patterns of light to support inferences about objects, surfaces, and actions you might take to interact with the environment, we must consider what light is and how it gets into your nervous system in the first place. The exercises in this chapter are all concerned with how to describe the physical nature of light and the way it behaves. We begin by investigating some simple properties of how light interacts with different kinds of matter (**Reflection, Refraction**, and **Diffraction** exercises) and how we can use diffraction in particular to examine the contents of different light sources via **Spectroscopy**. A key question we will try to answer in this section is this: What is physically different about lights that are different colors? Red, green, and blue lights all look different to us, but how do they actually differ from one another? We'll try to make the case that color is linked to a physical property of light called *wavelength*, which is a part of the wave model of light.

Take a look at Figure 1.1 and you'll see examples of light doing a bunch of different things: Light is being generated by the candle, it's bouncing off some surfaces, passing through others, and it even looks like in some cases it's getting stuck on surfaces without going anywhere afterwards. We're going to use some specific terms to describe each of these behaviors so that we have a common language for talking about the different things that light does.

Emission – Light can be produced by some objects that we'll call *sources*. In Figure 1.1, the candle is a source that is emitting light from the flame.

Absorption – Sometimes when light encounters a material, it stops. The physics of what happens after it stops is beyond the scope of our discussion, so for our purposes we're going to focus on the fact that absorption means light travels no further.

Reflection – Sometimes when light encounters a material, it bounces off. You are probably most used to thinking about reflection with regard to mirrored surfaces, but reflection happens when light encounters surfaces that don't look shiny to us, too. Indeed, the way we get to see most objects is by light from a source striking the object and reflecting towards our eyes afterwards. In Figure 1.1, the light emerging from the red disc at the bottom of the picture is reflecting in different directions after arriving at the disc from the source.

Refraction – When light travels through one type of material into another, it changes direction. In Figure 1.1, the crooked path light is taking as it moves through the tilted blue object is the result of this property of light.

DOI: 10.4324/9781032691169-2

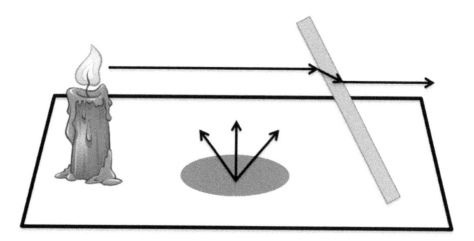

Figure 1.1 A cartoon depicting several of the things light can do when interacting with surfaces and objects in the environment. Light can be emitted from sources as in the candle at left, it can bend as it passes through different media like the prism at the right, and it can be both absorbed by surfaces and reflected from them as you see in the red spot in the middle. Illustration by the author.

Diffraction – Light bends around corners when it encounters them. This isn't depicted in Figure 1.1, but will turn out to be a very important way for us to make connections between different observations we can make to understand what color is in terms of physical properties of light.

Two Models of Light

Speaking of physical properties of light, I want to introduce two different ways to think about light as a physical stimulus that we will use throughout this section to understand what is happening in the different observations we will make: (1) Light is a *particle*, and (2) light is a *wave*. Each of these viewpoints offers useful ways to understand how vision works, and we'll use both of them to reason about what we see and why. Our goal in this chapter is to arrive at an understanding of color in terms of some part of one (or both) of these models. To elaborate on this, let's say more about these two models and how linking light to a specific physical description can help us draw conclusions about its nature.

Light Is a Particle

Our first model of light is very simple: To think about light as a particle, I want you to imagine a very small bullet or ping-pong ball flying straight through the air. This is our basic picture of what light is when we use this model. What does this get us in terms of reasoning about physical properties of light? A real ping-pong ball or bullet flying around like this must have some speed and it also must have a direction that it is moving in. There could be fast bullets and slow bullets, and they might fly in all different directions. We're going to say that all of our light bullets (or *photons*) have the same speed, but can fly in all directions just fine. Is there more that we can say about them? You could try imagining other ways that real particles like this could differ from one another (maybe their size, for example) and keep these ideas in mind when you see light do different things. Also, you have some expectations about what real bullets or ping-pong balls do when they hit some kind of surface, or move from one kind of material to another. Those expectations about particle behavior are also important ways to potentially link observations of light to physical properties.

Light Is a Wave

Our second model of light is also simple and involves another physical phenomena you likely have some experience with. To think about light as a wave, I want you to imagine actual waves of water in a lake, on the ocean, or in a small container holding some fluid. Another good way to have a picture of waves in mind is to think about a long rope being held by two people, with one of them shaking their end to make the rope go up and down. In both cases, we can see that waves also travel with some direction and with some speed (like our photons), but we have some new physical properties that we can think about, too.

For one thing, those waves we are imagining have a height to them: Waves can be tall, or they can be short. I'm going to call this the *amplitude* of the wave. What else can be different about different waves? Besides changing how tall the waves are, I hope you can also imagine that we could change how close together the peaks of those ripples are. Some waves could have lots of ripples close together, while others could have them spread far apart. I'm going to call this the *wavelength* of the wave.

There is another property I want you to think about next, mostly to get you thinking about linking a model of light to what light itself actually does. Besides shaking up and down with closely spaced or more distant ripples, the waves we create with a long piece of rope can shake in different orientations, too. That is, we could either shake the rope up and down, or we could shake it left-to-right and get a sideways wave. If we were feeling ambitious, we could also shake the rope at some sort of tilted angle to make a diagonally oriented wave. I'm going to call this property the *polarization* of the wave. Like the size of the bullets that we mentioned in the previous section, here is a property of this model that's easy for us to think about, but that we don't know (yet) how to link to some aspect of how light looks to us. The interesting part will be trying to make those connections so that we can arrive at a better understanding of light and how it interacts with our visual system.

Now we have to different ways to think about what light is in terms of simple physical phenomena you already have some intuitions about. We can imagine that light is a bunch of bullets flying straight through the air, or we can think about light as a bunch of waves sort of rippling through the air. Now that we've got some ideas in mind for what light is, let's get started observing what light *does*.

Absorption – How Does Light Get Absorbed by Different Materials?

Our goal in this first chapter is to get acquainted with light and different things that it does when it interacts with matter. We'll start by examining different kinds of light, by which I mean different colors of lights, and evaluating how an ordinary material (you!) absorbs these different lights (see Figure 1.2). Where we're heading is towards an understanding of what makes lights that look different to us physically different from one another, an understanding we'll try to reach by observing the behavior of light as a function of how it looks.

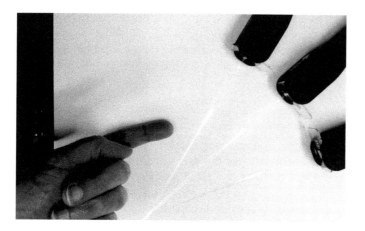

Figure 1.2 Laser pointers in three colors (red, green, and blue) alongside a finger that is ready to absorb some of the light emitted by these sources. Photo by the author.

Things you will need:

• Laser pointers in red, green, and blue.
• Your finger.

E.T. Phones Home, or How Red Light Is Absorbed by Your Finger

We'll begin with as simple a demonstration as I can think of: Take your red laser pointer, press the opening of it right against your finger and turn the thing on. My guess is that doing so led to something that looks a lot like the picture in Figure 1.3: Your finger

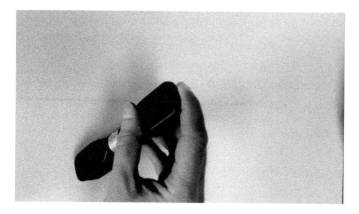

Figure 1.3 A red laser pointer held up against your finger should lead to a glowing red fingertip as the light mostly passes through your skin. Green and blue lasers held up against your finger should be much less interesting. In these cases, nearly all of the light is absorbed by the tissue in your finger. Photo by the author.

should be glowing red, which surely means something with regard to how your skin, muscle, bone, and blood did or did not absorb this kind of light. But why exactly does your finger look red under these circumstances?

You might have a few ideas about this. One idea might be that the red light from the laser is mostly just passing through your finger, exiting out the other side and heading for your eye until you see some red light. Another idea might be that your body's tissues and blood tend to be, well, red. Does this red color have less to do with the light and more to do with the stuff inside your finger? To test this out, let's see what happens if you replace the red laser with the green or blue one.

Green and Blue Light Absorption by Your Finger

When you replace the red laser with one of the other two, my guess is that it won't look nearly like that last picture. Instead, you will likely see nothing more than small amount of light escaping along the surface of your finger from the opening of the laser pointer. This suggests that it isn't just the case that any old bright light will do something to illuminate the red tissue and blood inside our finger to make it glow. Instead, this shows off that our finger soaks up some kinds of light more than others. Red light seems to mostly pass right through, while green and blue light seem to get stuck or absorbed once they hit this material.

This is a first hint that the differences in how lights look to us can be related to different things they will do when they encounter different objects and surfaces. For now, what we know is that light can look different in terms of something we call color and that this has something to do with whether or not light is absorbed when it strikes a material. Can we link this to any of the physical properties of light that we discussed in our particle and wave models of light? So far, I think it's not so easy to understand how we could do that. We don't have an obvious way to argue that different color lights must be particles of different size, for example. All we know is that there is something about color that affects absorption. Let's keep looking at different kinds of light behavior and see how we can think about color in particular, and light more generally, using our particle and wave models as a guide.

Reflection – How Does Light Bounce off of Surfaces?

Understanding how patterns of light are processed by the visual system begins by understanding how light behaves physically when it doesn't just get stuck to a surface. What else does light do when it encounters objects, surfaces, and materials in the environment, and how do we describe these behaviors? Can we use these descriptions to help us work out what light is and make predictions about what it will do in other circumstances? Understanding these behaviors will be very important for our understanding of how images are formed in the eye, a critical first step towards turning light from an external physical phenomenon into an internal perceptual phenomenon. Here, we'll examine the nature of *reflection*, which refers to the way light bounces off a surface, with two questions in mind: (1) Does reflection work differently for different kinds of light?; (2) How can we quantify the way light bounces off of a surface?

Things you will need (pictured in Figure 1.4):

- Laser pointers in red, green, and blue.
- Some small mirrors (~3" × 3", but size is not crucial).

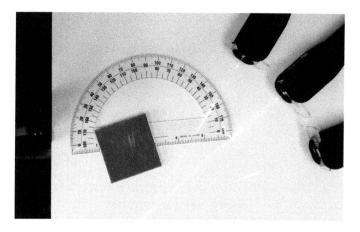

Figure 1.4 Red, green, and blue laser pointers (or LED lights), a protractor, and some hand mirrors are all you need to observe the Law of Reflection. Photo by the author.

- A protractor.
- A whiteboard and some dry-erase markers (pencil and paper will do too).

Does Reflection Work Differently for Different Colors of Light?

Our next question is to determine whether or not different kinds of lights (by which we mean different colors) reflect differently from one another. That is, if different lights come at a surface from the same direction, do they take different paths after they bounce off?

To find out, stand your mirror up on edge so that it is perpendicular to the whiteboard or paper you are working on. Mark a point on the paper that it is in the middle of the mirror and shine one of your lasers along the surface of your workspace so that it hits that point and bounces off of the mirror (this should yield a V-shaped path like you see at left in Figure 1.5). Trace this path with your marker or pencil, then replace the first laser you used with a different color. If you match the incoming path, does the new laser take a different outgoing path? You should be able to see that reflection works the same whether we're using a red, green, or blue laser.

How Can We Quantify the Path Light Will Take When It Reflects?

Our next step is to determine what path light takes after bouncing off of a surface, which we've just seen doesn't depend on the color of the light we're talking about. To do this, we'll use our protractor to make measurements of the incoming and outgoing paths light takes after bouncing off of our mirror.

Repeat the steps we described above (marking a point for your laser to reflect from and shining the light on the mirror so you can trace the path it makes), with one addition: Lightly trace the line at the bottom of the mirror (through the point you marked) so that you have a straight line representing the mirror on your work surface, the point where the light hit the mirror, and the V-shaped path the light took on the way into and away from the mirror. The lines you traced should make three different angles on the paper – One angle is in the middle of the V-shaped path you've traced. The other two angles are

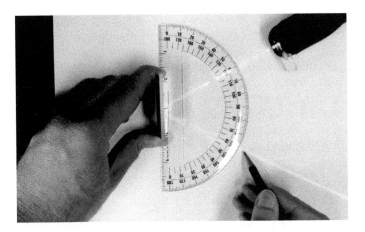

Figure 1.5 Measure the angles made by an incoming and outgoing ray of light as it bounces off of the surface of your mirror. Photo by the author.

between one of the lines making up that V and half of the line making up the mirror (one angle to the left of the V and another to the right of it). Use your protractor (see the right side of Figure 1.5) to measure how big those two angles are, then measure the angle inside the V as well.

You should find that the two angles flanking the V are the same. Try repeating these steps with a different incoming path for the light and confirm that whatever you do, those two angles stay equal across different incoming directions. You should also find that adding up all three angles gives you a total of 180 degrees.

This set of observations probably didn't hold too many surprises for you, but we should still talk carefully about what we saw. First of all, what did light do when it encountered a mirror? When we measure the various angles that light makes relative to the surface of a mirror on the way in and the way out, we should find that the angles between the mirror's surface and the incoming/outgoing rays of light will be equal. This *Law of Reflection* is usually described slightly differently in terms of what are called the *incident angles*, but the point is the same.

The fact that this behavior didn't turn out to depend on the color of light that you used means that once again it's not obvious how to build a bridge between either of our physical light models and color. Reflection thus doesn't seem to be terribly useful for understanding what color is in terms of a physical property of light. Still, this is a case where it's useful to see how a physical analog of light like our particle model helps us think about something light does with reference to something that another physical object (like a billiard ball) does under similar circumstances: Ricocheting a ball off of the side of a pool table will lead to the same change in direction as the one you just observed, which is a reassuring sign that it's meaningful to keep these kinds of physical models in mind as we explore light.

The observation that there is a simple lawful behavior governing reflection is also important because we can use this fact to calculate things that light is going to do and think about what follows from that calculation. Every time that light reflects off of a surface, we know that these angles we have examined have to be equal, and it doesn't matter what color the light is. Maybe this seems rather trivial to you, but it means that we have the ability to control the direction light is traveling as we see fit using mirrors, and we can use our understanding of the law to think through why we see some of the things that we do reflected in a mirrored surface.

In particular, we can even get fancy and talk about curved mirrors if we want. All we have to do is think about a curved surface as a collection of very small flat surfaces linked together. That way, we imagine that light hitting a particular spot on a curved mirror is really like hitting a very small flat mirror tilted to follow the curved surface. The formal name for that imaginary flat mirror is the *tangent* to the curved surface, and once you've found it, you can use the Law of Reflection to figure out where light is going to go after it bounces off a spoon, a ball bearing, or whatever you like.

Using the Law of Reflection to Plan a Path for Light

As a final challenge, try to use this fact about how light reflects to plan a path for a laser beam. On your work surface, choose a starting point for the light, an ending point where you want it to go, and a few other points in between that are places you want it to ricochet from on its way between the start and the end. Connect the dots between all these points to make a path from the start to the end, then use the equal-angles law you've just discovered to work out how a mirror at each midpoint needs to be positioned so that the light will follow the path you've drawn. Once you have lines for each mirror drawn on the paper, try putting mirrors at each location to see if the light goes where you intended (see Figure 1.6).

The big idea here is simple, but matters a great deal: We can predict where light will go once we understand the laws that govern its interaction with surfaces and materials. This allows us to both explain some basic phenomena related to how light moves through the environment on its way to our eye and also to manipulate light in predictable ways to achieve outcomes that require light to be in specific places. Despite how simple the Law of Reflection

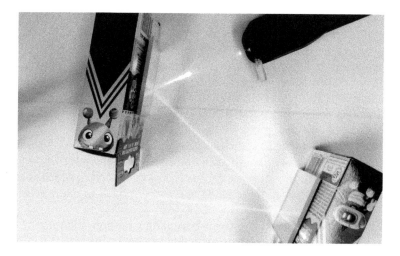

Figure 1.6 Knowing the Law of Reflection can make it possible for you to predict a complex path incorporating many reflections. Photo by the author.

is, most people find it difficult to reason correctly about what will and won't be visible in a mirror (Bertamini & Soranzo, 2018). This is an interesting case in which cognitive and perceptual biases interact with one another such that our intuitions about mirrors often don't match the real paths that light takes as it bounces off of surfaces in the environment.

We will continue exploring geometric optics in the next section by examining the nature of refraction. In this next exercise, light will neither get stuck, nor bounce off of a surface, but instead pass through one kind of material and into another.

Refraction – What Happens When Light Passes from One Medium to Another?

If we're considering a material that is transparent or translucent, light won't just bounce off of the surface of this medium but will instead pass through the surface and into the material. Along the way, it will most likely change direction or *refract* as it crosses the boundary between two different kinds of stuff. Refraction happens at the boundary of any two different substances, including water, air, and various solid materials like plastic or glass. In this exercise, we'll ask one of the same questions about refraction that we asked about reflection: Does it happen differently for different kinds of light?

Things you will need (pictured in Figure 1.7):

- Laser pointers in red, green, and blue.
- A set of acrylic prisms: biconvex, biconcave, and straight.
- A straightedge.

Observing Refraction for Different Lights with a Triangular Prism

Begin by placing your straight prism (the one with the triangular tip) onto your work surface (a whiteboard or piece of paper). It will probably be useful to put some tape under it to keep it in place, but this isn't necessary. Pick one of your lasers (let's say the green one)

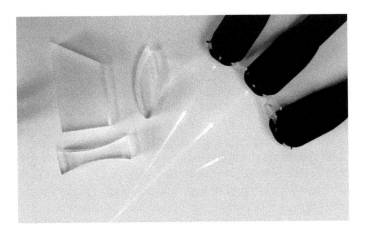

Figure 1.7 Red, green, and blue laser pointers (or LED lights), acrylic prisms, and a protractor will allow you to measure the nature of refraction as light passes from one medium to another. Photo by the author.

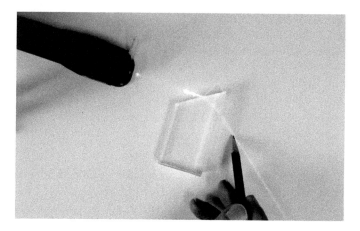

Figure 1.8 You should be able to observe light bending as it passes through the two tilted surfaces of the triangular portion of a prism like this. Note that some of the light is also reflected by the surface at the top, in accordance with the Law of Reflection. Photo by the author.

and shine it across the surface so that it enters into one of the sides of the triangular tip and exits out of the other one. You should be able to see the incoming and outgoing rays tilted in different directions on the opposite sides of the prism. Trace both of these lines with a pencil or marker (see Figure 1.8).

You will probably notice that at some angles, there is also a bit of the incoming ray that is reflected off of the first surface of the prism. One thing to play around with here is figuring out when that reflection stops as you change the incoming angle between the light and the prism surface. If you like, add a dotted line to show when that reflection appears to stop happening.

Once you've done both of these steps, repeat these steps with the remaining lasers. Critically, match up the incoming path for each of the other two colors, and see how closely the outgoing path matches what you traced for the other two. It will likely only be a subtle difference, but you should be able to see that the outgoing red, green, and blue paths are in fact just a little bit different.

Observing Refraction for Different Lights with Convex/Concave Prisms

We can look at the difference in refraction as a function of the color of our light sources using prisms with a different shape as well. Let's begin by using a convex prism (this one has sides that bulge outwards) to measure the focal length of this curved prism or *lens*. To do this, fix the convex prism to your work surface using tape and point your laser straight at the very middle of the lens. You should see the light pass straight through the lens without bending. Go ahead and trace this line onto your work surface. Next, keeping your light pointed straight at the lens, slide it a short way up or down – the incoming light ray should still be perpendicular to the lens (keep the ray parallel to the direction you started with), but, as you move the laser vertically, you will see the outgoing light ray turning more and more sharply downwards towards the middle of the lens. Trace a few of these outgoing rays (see Figure 1.9), and make a mark at the point where they cross paths with each other. This crossing is the focal point for this lens and the distance between the prism and this point is the focal length.

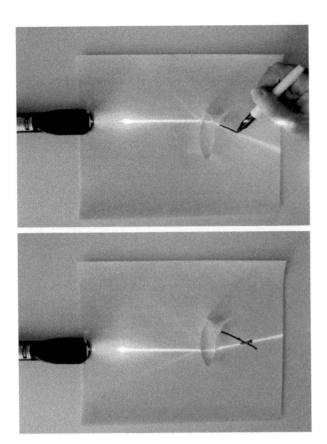

Figure 1.9 Curved lenses will focus light rays that are perpendicular to their axis at a locus we will refer to as the focal length. Photo by the author.

Repeat these steps with the other two laser colors, and see how the focal length compares across light sources. Again, though this may be a little subtle, you should be able to see that the red, green, and blue lasers have slightly different focal lengths.

We can try out this same observation with our concave lens (the prism with sides that are sunken in). Repeat these same steps, but note that, as you move the light source vertically, the light rays now bend upwards away from the middle of the prism. This means that our outgoing light rays will still cross paths, but at a point that is on the same side of the prism as the laser. With this in mind, find the focal length of this prism using all three lenses, and see how different these are from one another.

Compared to reflection, refraction thus appears to be a phenomenon that affects different colors of light differently. Specifically, blue light appears to bend more than green light as it passes into this new medium, and green light bends more than red.

This is getting more interesting – we now have a property of light besides absorption that has something to do with color! Let's return to our physical models of light for a moment: Why does this happen? Can we think about the way a particle or a wave might behave if we asked it pass from one medium into another? If we're really thinking about a small particle like a bullet, my guess is that it's a little tough to imagine that projectile changing course by very much if we did something like firing it into a pool of water. I've also watched enough corny action movies with underwater sequences to tell you that the paths bullets take under these circumstances sure seem to stay pretty straight. The particle model of light may not be our best bet for understanding this phenomenon. Instead, if we consider how a wave would act under the same circumstances, we can think through how this bending or turning might take place. To do so, we need to focus on two things regarding waves in other physical situations – (1) A wave is an extended phenomenon. That is, waves aren't like little bullets that are small and compact. Instead, they're like a long ridge or ripple that extends across some amount of space; (2) Waves can move faster or slower in different mediums (air vs. water vs. gelatin). While this second property is true for particles too, the first one is not.

What do these two facts imply about what will happen to a wave that passes from one medium (like air) into another (like the acrylic in your lenses)? Because waves are extended things, If part of a wave encounters a new medium and slows down a bit when it gets there, the part of it that hasn't entered yet will still be going faster. But what happens to something if one side of it is going faster than the other? If you've ever had one side of your car hit an icy or slushy spot in the road, you know the rather scary answer to this question: You start turning!

This amount of this turning turns out to have a law that goes with it, much like the Law of Reflection. We can calculate how much a given light will turn if we know some things about the two materials it passes through and the angle it makes on the way in. The specific relationship we need is called Snell's Law, and it includes terms for the angles light makes before and after passing through a new medium as well as for the speed of light in each medium. Those angles are marked θ1 and θ2 in Figure 1.10, and the terms that correspond to the speed of light in each medium are marked n1 and n2.

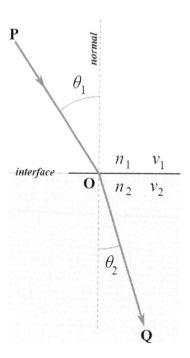

Figure 1.10 A diagram of light refracting as it passes from one medium with an index of refraction of n1 into another with a refraction index of n2. Snell's Law is an equation that describes how these indices are related to the two angles that characterize the light's path on both sides of the surface between the two substances.

But where does color figure into this? This equation doesn't obviously help us understand how color relates to either those angles we use in Snell's Law or those 'n' numbers. I am going to leave you in mild suspense for the moment, because we have a rather fun reveal coming up. For now, what I want to get across is that we now have an interesting physical phenomenon involving light and more importantly the color of light, which means we may be getting closer to understanding what color is in terms of our different models. The fact that we could only explain refraction by appealing to our wave model is potentially an important hint that we'll need the properties that accompany thinking of light as a wave to understand the nature of color. Also, we see yet again that light obeys some simple physical laws that we can use to make predictions about where light will go, which in turn helps us understand why we see what we see when light passes through different materials.

Diffraction – How Does Light Behave When It Encounters Corners?

Things you will need:

- Laser pointers (red, green, and blue – at minimum use red and blue to maximize wavelength difference).
- A diffraction grating. The "Rainbow Peephole" pictured in Figure 1.11 can be bought in bulk very inexpensively.
- A strand of hair (I know this seems a little gross, but still).
- An aluminum baking tray.
- A small plastic Duplo brick or other small object (~2" to a side).

Watching Water Waves Bend around Corners

The phenomena we're about to observe are all consequences of *diffraction* or the bending of light around corners. Diffraction is a property of waves more generally, so this will be a

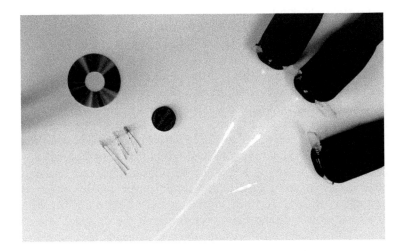

Figure 1.11 Red, green, and blue laser points, some LEDs with a button battery (a CR2032 or similar will work), a small diffraction grating, a pocket spectroscope, and a strand of hair will allow you to observe diffraction. Photo by the author.

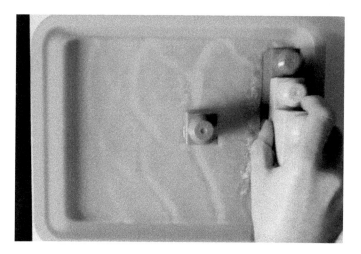

Figure 1.12 Water waves will bend around a small object placed in their path. If light is also a wave, it should do the same thing. In this image, you can see how the single wavefront in the middle turns into two waves that cross one another at the left. Photo by the author.

good opportunity to consider our wave model of light more closely in our efforts to link color to some specific physical property of light. Remember, the point of using a model like this is to guide our thinking based on our intuitions about the parts of the model. To help us think about what we see light waves do during diffraction, we're going to begin by watching water waves diffract first.

To do this, fill your aluminum tray with water, and place the brick I mentioned above roughly in the middle of the tray. Now, use something like a ruler or other flat object that is about as wide as the tray to make waves in the water by moving the ruler up and down in the water at one end (see Figure 1.12). This should allow you to see roughly flat wavefronts move across the water and then bend around the corners of the brick. There are two important things I want you to look for and think about in this water-wave version of diffraction: (1) Try making the ripples have a shorter wavelength (the space between crests of neighboring waves) by moving your ruler up and down more rapidly. It may be a little hard to see, but I hope you can make out that there is more bending around the corner of the brick when you shake the ruler more slowly; (2) Because those waves are bending around the opposite sides of the brick, waves from the two sides of the brick will end up meeting each other after they travel further along in the tray.

The first observation is important because it tells us that the amount of bending during diffraction is directly related to wavelength. Explaining why this is true is beyond the scope of this book, so for now we'll just take that observation on face value and remember that we saw it happen: A shorter wavelength meant *less* bending. The second observation is important because it helps us make a prediction about something that ought to happen if light also behaves like a wave under these circumstances – light waves bending around the two sides of a small object should meet each other on the opposite side of the object from the source. This matters a lot because when waves meet, they *interfere* with each other. Again, you can probably rely on some intuitions you have about water waves to help you imagine what interference means. If two large water waves happen to run into one another so that their crests meet, the two waves add up to yield a crest that's much higher than either of the two starting peaks. We call this *constructive interference*, and the opposite phenomenon is called *destructive interference*, which occurs when the crest of one wave meets the trough of another. In this latter case, the two waves still add up, but the combination of a crest and a trough effectively cancels out the height of either wave, leading to water that's nearly flat. The reason I'm asking you to step through all this by thinking about water is that now we can make a prediction about what we should see if light waves are meeting up and interfering with one another after diffracting around a small object. Light should add up to be either brighter or darker than what we started with! Let's take a look and see if this actually happens in our next set of observations.

Watching Light Waves Bend around a Strand of Hair

Remember, if water waves bend around a small object, then we should be able to get light waves to bend around something, too. Because light waves have such a small wavelength, however, it turns out we need to use a much narrower object than our brick. To observe diffraction with a laser pointer, we'll make light waves bend around a strand of human hair that we tape across the opening of our laser pointer. Make sure you have a strand that is long enough to cross the opening of your laser and secure it tightly across on both sides.

With that strand of hair in place, turn on the laser pointer and shine the beam onto a white piece of paper (something more matte and less shiny will make it easier to see). What you should see is a pattern of light and dark bars stretching out horizontally (see Figure 1.13). What's going on? The light waves bending around the hair are indeed interfering with one another the same way that the water waves bending around the Duplo brick did. In some places, the peak of one wave meets the peak of another, leading to a larger amplitude/intensity of light and a bright spot on the paper. In neighboring places,

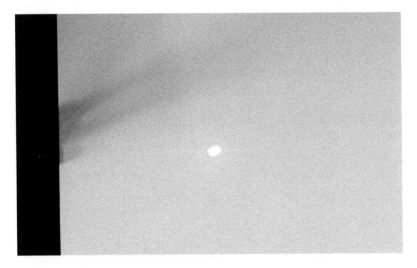

Figure 1.13 The light waves that bend around the strand of hair meet on the other side of the hair, leading to constructive and destructive interference that we can see as either bright stripes or dark stripes. Photo by the author.

the peak of one wave meets the trough of another, leading to the two waves canceling out and a dark spot on the paper.

I want to pause for a second to point out how neat this is. We had a guess that light might act like waves, we checked out what a different kind of wave did under conditions where diffraction happened, and we used that observation to guess what light should do in the same kind of situation. The fact that we were right demonstrates that this wave model of light is indeed a good physical description of what light is that helps us predict its behavior. In this case, it would be tough to explain this observation solely with the particle model of light, so it matters that we have an alternative model in mind.

So light diffracts, and when it does it can end up self-interfering to produce this interesting stripey pattern. That wasn't the only thing we knew about diffraction based on our observations of water waves, though, so let's move on to thinking about wavelength and the amount of diffraction we observe from different kinds of light.

Using a Diffraction Grating to Compare Diffraction for Different Colors

This set of observations relies on using an inexpensive optical device called a diffraction grating. A diffraction grating like the Rainbow Peephole pictured in Figure 1.14 is a thin film with many narrow scratches etched into it. Each of those scratches gives light a new set of corners to bend around, making these excellent tools for bending different colors of light to see how they behave. You can look through the peephole at different light sources (something we'll do next in the **Spectroscopy** exercise) but here I want you to shine your different lasers through the peephole to see how different colors of light spread out when they diffract (A reminder: Never shine a laser pointer directly into your eyes!).

For each of your three lasers, point them at a surface some fixed distance away (this can be a wall or a piece of paper) and turn them on with the diffraction grating in front of the laser's opening. You should see that instead of a single laser pointer dot the diffraction grating yields an array of dots. Measure the distance between these dots for each color – you should find that red is the most spread out, followed by green, then blue (see the images in Figure 1.14).

What is especially neat about this is that not only are we seeing that different colors of light diffract by different amounts, but now we can link this to a property of waves by comparing what we see here to what we saw with the water waves in our aluminum tray. In the

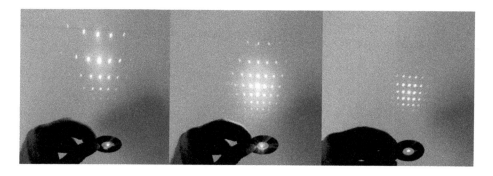

Figure 1.14 Light will spread out by different amounts after passing through a diffraction grating depending on what color it is. This allows us to link the color of light to the wavelength of light waves. Photos by the author.

case of the water waves, a shorter wavelength led to less bending around an object. Now that we're looking at light, we see that different colors of light bend by different amounts when they pass through the slits in the diffraction grating. This means that the physical difference between our laser pointers of different color must be the wavelength, with blue light having the shortest wavelength, green the next shortest, and red the longest. This connection between the physical properties of a wave and the perceptual property of color is what we were trying to establish in this chapter and here we are!

With this conclusion in hand, we can look back at what we saw in our previous observations of refraction and revisit some of what we saw light do as it obeyed Snell's Law. Remember that this was another case in which the color of light affected the outcome – red light bent the least as it passed through different materials, and blue light bent the most. Now we know that color implies something about wavelength, so we can reframe those observations by saying that long wavelengths bend the least during refraction and short wavelengths bend the most. Does this help us understand more about the nature of refraction? What I can tell you now is that wavelength does indeed sneak into Snell's Law in a way I didn't tell you about before. Those refractive indices (the "n's" in the equation) aren't the same for all kinds of light – the specific value of "n" that you need to calculate refraction depends on wavelength and tells you what the speed of light is in each material for that kind of light. This may not mean a ton to you at present, but it's a neat way to see how understanding more about the nature of a model we use to describe light helps us get deeper insights into what's happening.

Knowing that wavelength and color are tied together this way is thus an important first step towards understanding further observations of light under different circumstances and also offers the chance to develop a description of light that is more precise than just naming colors "red" or "green" or "blue." To help you get a sense of what that description looks like, we'll close this section by using diffraction to observe the ingredients of different light sources and further explore the relationship between wavelength and color.

Spectroscopy – Examining the Contents of Light Using Diffraction

We saw in our previous exercise (the **Diffraction** lab) that light will bend or diffract by different amounts through a slit as a function of its wavelength. Light with a smaller wavelength (more blue) will bend less than light with a longer wavelength (more red). The light we see from most sources is a mixture of light waves with different intensities and different wavelengths, and diffraction provides us with a simple means of spreading those light waves apart so we can observe the contents in a particular light source. This process is called *spectroscopy* and has applications in chemistry, astronomy, and many other disciplines. Here (see Figure 1.15), we will use it to build some intuitions about the lights in your surroundings and identify *metameric* colors. This term refers to lights/colors that are physically different from one another, but look the same to us due to the properties of our visual system. Figure 1.15

Things you will need:

- A spectroscope (not totally necessary, but nice to have and not too expensive).
- A rainbow peephole or other diffraction grating.
- LEDs of different colors.
- A button battery (CR232 or similar).

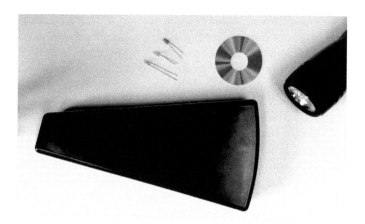

Figure 1.15 A spectroscope, a diffraction grating, LEDs, and some other light sources allow you to use diffraction to measure the ingredients of light sources. Photo by the author.

Basic Spectroscopy with a Diffraction Grating and an LED

We'll begin by observing some light sources that are safe to look at directly (unlike our lasers) and vary in their color. LEDs are a cheap and convenient light source that we can illuminate easily with a button battery. Just pinch the leads of your LED around the button battery and the LED should light up – if it doesn't, flip the leads around and you should be all set. Once the LED is lit up, take a look at it through your diffraction grating. Much like the spread out array of laser pointer dots we observed in the **Diffraction** lab, you should see many copies of the LED spread out into a similar array of colored streaks. What's more, those streaks should have a rainbow-like quality to them – different colors of light should be spread out in a smear radiating out from the middle of the array (see Figure 1.16). Take note of what colors you see and how bright they look to you (use the ROYGBIV spectrum to write down some subjective numbers of intensity for each color, for example). Make sure to look at LEDs that are different colors and compare what you see. Figure 1.16

Here I'm showing you what I can see with a white LED flashlight. Note that even though the light looks white in the very center of the picture, we can see red, yellow, green, and blue very clearly as the light with different wavelengths spreads out through the diffraction grating. This is an important indicator that the color you see is not a perfect indicator of everything that is in a light source.

Now let's use your spectroscope to look at some more lights. Remember to never look directly at lasers, the sun, or other extremely bright light sources (welding arcs, e.g.) without eye protection. Instead, use your spectroscope to look at different light sources around you that are different colors and see what wavelengths are present and absent from different lights.

An important thing to check out with your spectroscope is the phenomenon of *meta-merism*. Lights can have different wavelength ingredients but look identical to us because of how our visual system responds to light as a function of wavelength. To see this, find a few different lights that all look "white" to you: a white flashlight, white fluorescent tubes, and sunlight shining on a white piece of paper are all fine examples to use. Though all of

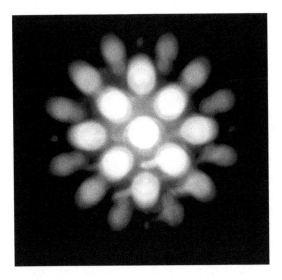

Figure 1.16 Through a diffraction grating, light sources spread out into a smeared spectrum of colors that shows off the different wavelengths of light that are part of the light in question. Photo by the author.

these are white as far as your vision is concerned, you should see that these have very different spectra: While sunlight will look like a continuous rainbow streak, for example, an LED flashlight that looks white will probably have strong spectral lines at red, green, and blue with gaps in between (see Figure 1.17).

Try to record a few different versions of "white" to see how different they can be. While you're at it, you may want to compare different versions of "red" or "green" to keep track of how variable these colors can be, too. Comparing what you get from electronic displays like your phone or a monitor to what you get from colors illuminated by sunlight (a bright

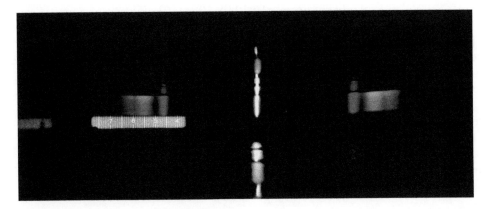

Figure 1.17 A spectroscope accomplishes the same feat as our diffraction gratings but often includes a scale for measuring wavelength and a more convenient display. Photo by the author.

blue patch of paint) should lead to some pretty clear differences. Wavelength clearly has a lot to do with the colors we see, but the colors we see are not perfect indicators of the wavelengths in the light we observe.

Besides remembering this fact for later, we can also use our spectroscopic observations to start thinking about a way to continue being as precise as possible when talking about light. Specifically, how could we translate these patterns of stripes that we see into a more formal description of different kinds of light? We've already established that different colors of light differ from one another in terms of their *wavelength*. If we're sticking with our wave model of light, we can also make another simple connection between another physical property of a wave and a perceptual property of light: Light of any wavelength can sometimes be bright and sometimes be faint, which is related to the *amplitude* of light, or the height of the wave that we're keeping in mind. A good description of light should include both of these pieces of information. We need to describe what wavelengths of light are present in a stimulus, and we should also describe how strong light is at each wavelength. I'm going to suggest that this means we could describe light using a list, which we'll call a *spectrum*. This word can refer to the kind of numerical list we're about to make, but it can also refer to the actual pattern of light and dark stripes you see when you spread out the different wavelengths of light that are present in a mixture of inputs. The key is understanding how we translate between the two.

Our numerical list will have an entry for each integer wavelength in the range of visible light (which includes light with wavelengths between 400nm and 700nm), and the magnitude of the number that we put in each place will tell us the strength of the light at that wavelength. Let's say a value of zero means that there's no light at that wavelength, while larger values (say 100, in arbitrary units) means that we have quite a lot of light at that wavelength. A generic light spectrum might look like this, if we just want to use symbols as placeholders for the wavelengths we'll include:

$$\text{Light spectrum} = [\lambda_1 \lambda_2 \lambda_3 \lambda_4 ... \lambda_n]$$

But a specific spectrum might look like this once we measure the intensity of light at different wavelengths:

$$\text{Light spectrum} = [0\ 10\ 98\ 10\ ...\ 50]$$

In both cases, the big deal is that we have a way of recording exactly what kind of light we are seeing, and use what we understand about waves, particles, reflection, refraction, and diffraction, to start thinking about what happens when light starts to interact both with objects in the environment and with our nervous system. With regard to the environment, our visual system's intuitive understanding of how reflection and refraction work contribute to the way we assess some objects as being made of things like metal or other shiny stuff (Fleming, 2017), glass (Todd & Norman, 2019) or looking soft and pliable vs. hard and brittle (Schmid & Doerschner, 2018). In our next chapter, we're going to take our first step inward by examining how patterns of light in the world become patterns of light in our eye, a process called *image formation*.

References

Bertamini, M., & Soranzo, A. (2018). Reasoning about visibility in mirrors: A comparison between a human observer and a camera. *Perception, 47*(8), 821–832. https://doi.org/10.1177/0301006618781088

Fleming, R. W. (2017). Material perception. *Annual Review of Vision Science, 3*, 365–388. https://doi.org/10.1146/annurev-vision-102016-061429

Schmid, A. C., & Doerschner, K. (2018). Shatter and splatter: The contribution of mechanical and optical properties to the perception of soft and hard breaking materials. *Journal of Vision, 18*(1), 14. https://doi.org/10.1167/18.1.14

Todd, J. T., & Norman, J. F. (2019). Reflections on glass. *Journal of Vision, 19*(4), 26. https://doi.org/10.1167/19.4.26

2 Image Formation in the Eye

For us to use light to measure appearance with our visual system, we have to get patterns of light into our nervous system from the outside world. In this set of exercises, we'll examine *image formation*, which is the first step in this process. Image formation refers to the way in which light from the environment is projected into the eye, ideally preserving the spatial layout of light across a visual scene and providing sufficient detail for us to recognize textures, objects, and people. The human eye achieves this through an optical set-up that we will explore by building a kind of model eye called a *pinhole camera*. By building one and observing the images formed with it (**Pinhole Optics**) we can see how the geometric optics principles we covered in the previous chapter help us understand how the parts of the eye help us obtain high-quality images on the retina. The quality of those images can be disrupted by conditions like near-sightedness (also known as *myopia*) however, and we'll use some modified versions of our pinhole camera to see the basis of this common visual impairment and explore how to correct it (**Correcting Myopia**). Finally, one noteworthy feature of pinhole optics is the formation of an inverted image. Our last exercise in this section (**Observing the Inverted Retina**) gives us a chance to see, with a simple optical set-up, that our own retinal image is inverted (Figure 2.1).

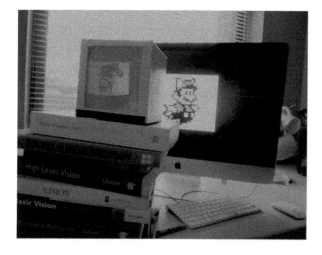

Figure 2.1 Image formation in a small camera obscura. Photo by the author.

DOI: 10.4324/9781032691169-3

Pinhole Optics – Using a Model Eye to Explore Image Formation

Patterns of light in the world become patterns of light in your nervous system via the formation of an image on the retina. Your eye is an optical device with anatomical features that support image formation (Wade & Finger, 2001), which we'll explore here by building a pinhole camera. The pinhole camera is an unsung hero of the photography world with some remarkable properties given how simple it is (Young, 1971). This cardboard camera will serve as a model system with parts that are analogues of some structures in the human eye. By exploring how the image that is projected on our model retina changes as we alter parts of the pinhole camera, we can understand how the anatomy of the eye contributes to good image formation in human vision (Figure 2.2).

Things you will need, as pictured in Figure 2.2:

- A small box. Bakery boxes that are ~8cm–10cm to a side are ideal.
- A biconvex lens with a focal length close to the box size.
- A small amount of tracing paper. You only need a piece big enough to cover one of the faces of the box.
- Electrical tape (though cellophane tape will do).
- Scissors.
- An LED.
- A button battery (CR232 or similar).

Building a Basic Pinhole Camera

Your first step is to put together the box, and add (1) a pupil to one side that will let light into the box's interior and (2) a viewing screen on the opposite side so that we can see how light is projected onto the rear surface of the camera. Begin by folding up your box and cutting a large square hole out of one of the faces. Leave enough room (1cm or so) around the border so that you have room to attach some tape there. Also, don't cut into either the top flap or the bottom of the box for this step. This will make it harder to affix

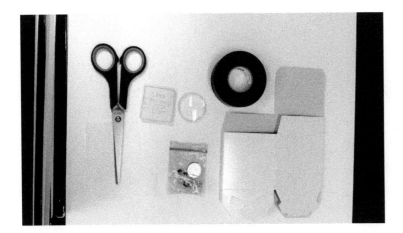

Figure 2.2 We can build a model eye from a small cardboard box, some tracing paper, and a lens. Photo by the author.

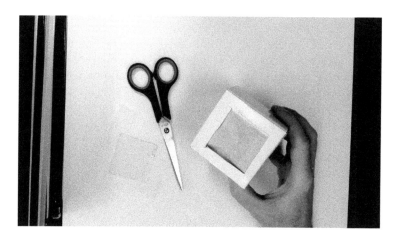

Figure 2.3 Begin by cutting out a square of your box so that you can replace it with a translucent viewing screen as depicted here. Photo by the author.

the tracing paper that we want to use as a projection screen. Continue by cutting out a square from your sheet of tracing paper to cover the hole you have just made. You can attach it either to the inside or outside of the box, but I find that using the inside tends to make the construction a little nicer. Pro tip: Use the cardboard square you cut out of the cardboard box to get the size of the tracing paper right (Figure 2.3).

Now that we have a way to see the patterns of light formed in our camera, we need to add an opening for the light to come in. Do this by poking a hole right in the middle of the side of the box *opposite* your viewing screen. This will allow light to come into this small hole and stream across the box until it strikes the tracing paper at the back of the camera. Use a pencil or another fairly small instrument to make this hole (Figure 2.4).

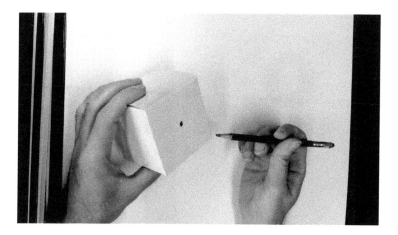

Figure 2.4 Add a small aperture to the side of your box opposite the viewing screen. Make this opening fairly small (we'll enlarge it later). Photo by the author.

Finally, use your electrical or cellophane tape to seal up any of the box's seams that aren't shut tight. Your goal in doing this is to minimize how much light can get in at the edges of the box, which will improve your image quality. It's not going to ruin things if you can't get the camera completely sealed up, but the more light-tight you can make it, the better.

At this point, let's take a moment to draw some parallels between this little pinhole camera and the image formation device you have in your head (the eye). As simple as the design of this cardboard device is, we can already make some connections between our model and the real thing. Remember: The goal of having a model we can manipulate is to give you a sense of the function of the different parts of the eye by having you make some observations after making changes to different parts of the model. We can start by linking the structures in our model to the structures in a real eye.

The Sclera – If you look at your own eye in a mirror, one of the main things you will see is the white orb of the eye itself. That tissue is called the *sclera*. There isn't a great deal to say about the sclera in terms of image formation because it primarily serves to protect the inner workings of the eye and also to maintain a consistent eye shape. This is important work, however, and we will see later on in this section that there are properties of the sclera that turn out to matter quite a bit when we are trying to get patterns of light onto the retina. Presently, though, I want you to think about the sclera as a necessary structure so that we have an eye at all. In our pinhole camera model of the eye, our artificial sclera is the cardboard box you assembled.

The Pupil – To continue considering parts of the eye we can see by looking in a mirror, let's think about the pupil, which is the black dot at the center of your eye. You probably already knew this, but this is the opening through which light passes to get from the outside world to the inside of your eye. An important feature of the pupil in a real eye is that it is capable of changing in size, due to the contraction or relaxation of muscles that surround the pupil in the *iris*, which is the pigmented donut-shaped region immediately surrounding the pupil. Shining light on the pupil will make it smaller, while removing that light will make it larger (see Figure 2.5).

If you want to play an interesting trick with this effect, you can try shining a light right on the border between the pupil and the iris. If the very edge of the light falls onto the pupil, the pupil will constrict so that the light is no longer shining on it. This means that

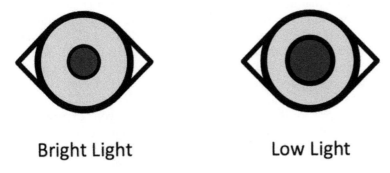

Bright Light   **Low Light**

Figure 2.5 The pupil dilates when in darkness and constricts when exposed to bright light. Illustration by the author.

the pupil is now in relative darkness so it will expand again until it hits the edge of the light, upon which it will shrink again. The result is that the pupil sort of bounces back and forth, or *oscillates* in size under these conditions.

This dynamic behavior from the human pupil is in stark contrast to the pupil in our model, which is the hole that we have poked into the center of one of the faces of the box. All models have limitations, however, and this is one of the limitations of our pinhole camera. Even so, our cardboard sclera and simplistic pupil will allow us to learn some important things. This depends critically on being able to observe the images being formed in our camera, which brings me to the last structure in our pinhole camera that we need to link to the human eye.

The Retina – Now we come to a part of the human eye that you can't see just by looking in a mirror. At the very back of your eyeball is a thin layer of tissue called the retina, which is where patterns of light are turned into electrical impulses that are sent to the rest of your visual system. We will of course have a lot more to say about the nature of this process in later sections, but for now the main idea to keep in mind is that this tissue is where we would like our image to end up. To say this more clearly, patterns of light in the world will become patterns of light on the retina based on how image formation proceeds in the eye. This is important to emphasize because the starting point for our visual processing is the arrangement of light on the retina. To start thinking about qualities of our visual experience, we will thus need to think carefully about the different things that are happening to light rays on their path from the outside world to the back of our eye. In your cardboard pinhole camera, the artificial retina is the translucent sheet of tracing paper you taped over the square hole opposite the pinhole. Obviously, this is a major deviation from how a real eye is put together, but we need to be able to see what's going on.

Testing the Pinhole Camera

Having established links between the pinhole camera and the eye, and with the basic camera now complete, your next step is to ensure that you can see patterns of light on the viewing screen. We can check this quickly using our button battery and an LED of any color.

Begin by making a "firefly" from the LED and your button battery by pinching the LED leads on either side of the battery. This should make the LED light up, but, if it doesn't, try flipping the battery over and giving it another shot. Once it's shining, hold it right in front of the pinhole, and look at the viewing screen. This should yield an image of the LED on the tracing paper that most likely looks like a fuzzy red dot (Figure 2.6).

Move the LED up and down or side to side, and observe the effect on the position and motion of the dot on the viewing screen (remember, this is our model retina). You should see that the image moves in the opposite direction than the LED itself is moving. Also try varying the distance between the pinhole and the LED and observe what happens on the screen. You should see that increasing the distance makes the image smaller while decreasing the distance will make it bigger.

Once you confirm that you can see the image of the LED well on your camera, look at a more complex scene. The trick to observing a good image is to point the pinhole at a bright scene while keeping the viewing screen in relative darkness. If it's a bright day outside, pointing the camera towards a window while standing in a dim or dark room tends to work very well. If your viewing circumstances are different and don't permit this, you can also try covering your head and the camera with a dark blanket or sheet while making

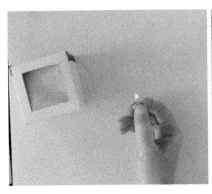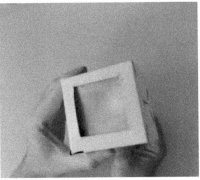

Figure 2.6 You should be able to see a small light source like your LED on the viewing screen if you hold it in front of the pinhole you made on the other side of the box. Photo by the author.

sure the pinhole is uncovered and pointing towards the scene you wish to view. Either way, hopefully you will be able to see a full scene projected onto the viewing screen. This is all you need to turn light fields in the environment into 2D projections! The simplicity of the pinhole camera means that you can really make one out of just about anything (see Cabe, 2003, for instructions on how to make a ping-pong ball version) and sometimes "accidental pinholes" become evident when light shines through small openings onto a surface. The gaps between the leaves on a tree, curtains that don't quite close all the way, and even the tiny holes in cookies and crackers (Cabe, 2018): all can serve as natural pinhole cameras under the right conditions. For our purposes, this little box is a good place to start thinking about what else must be happening in our eye and our visual brain to start working with 2D projections of light.

An important observation to make about this image is that it should be upside-down and flipped left-to-right: The sky should be at the bottom of the viewing screen and the ground should be at the top. This is a direct consequence of how light gets from the outside world to the viewing screen. Because your camera is sealed up carefully, the only way light can get from an object in the environment to the viewing screen is by passing through the pinhole in the front of the camera. This means that light from the top of a visual scene passes through the pinhole on a downward trajectory, ending up at the bottom of the screen (see the image in Figure 2.7). Light from the bottom of a visual scene passes through on an upward trajectory, ending up at the top of the screen. Thus, patterns of light in the outside world end up reversed after they pass through the pinhole, solely because of the geometry of the world and the imaging system (Figure 2.7).

You may find this a bit troubling: Is it a problem that these images are upside-down? You already might have been wondering how closely this model approximates what's going on in your own eye, and this outcome may inspire some doubt. Does your eyeball really have inverted images in it? Hopefully seeing this happen with a simple model is a powerful indicator that this feature of image formation is a basic consequence of the physics of light and the geometry of the eye. Hold this thought, though, because we'll return to it later on in this section with another set of observations.

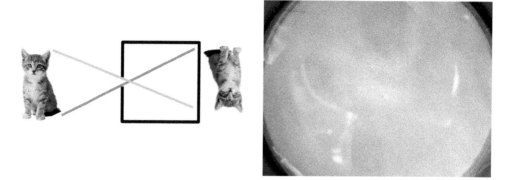

Figure 2.7 You should also be able to observe a full scene projected onto your viewing screen (see right) as long as the scene is bright and you can keep the viewing screen in relative darkness. That image will be upside-down and reversed left-to-right, however, due to the paths light must take between the outside world and the box through the pinhole opening (left). Illustration and photo by the author.

Improving Image Quality by Adding a Lens to the Pinhole Camera

The image you can see with this basic camera is going to be quite dim which is not ideal. It would be nice if we could make it easier to see what's happening in the world via our projected image, and one simple way to do so is to try making the pinhole opening bigger to let more light in. Continue by altering your camera in exactly this way: Widen that original pinhole (which should have been about the width of a pencil) so that it is about the size of a nickel or a quarter (approx. 2.5cm should do).

This rather clunky modification of our model eyeball is analogous to the changes in pupil size that we described previously: If there isn't very much light in the environment, the pupil can dilate to allow more light into the eye – if there is a great deal of light, it can contract to limit the amount of light that gets in. We haven't built a mechanism for varying the size of our model pupil, so poking a larger hole will have to do. Does letting more light into the camera in this fashion help us get a brighter and better image on the retina? Once you've widened your model pupil, take a look at a real-world scene again, and you should find that it is a lot brighter. This is accompanied by an unfortunate side-effect, however: The image is brighter, but also blurrier. We've made our image more intense, but we've also incurred a potentially serious cost (Figure 2.8).

Why should this be the case? Let's think again about the issue of how light can get from the world outside the camera to the viewing screen. Inverted images resulted from light having limited paths between the world and the screen, and this tradeoff between brightness and blurriness is also a direct result of that same fact. To understand why, let's simplify the situation we've created by widening the model pupil in a different way. Let's say that, to compensate for your pinhole camera image being too dim, you chose to make a second hole a short distance away from the first instead of widening the pupil. The problem with your dim image is that not enough light was getting into the camera, so a second hole seems like a perfectly fine solution, right? Two holes = double the light! But what does this mean for the image formed on the back of the viewing screen (Figure 2.9)?

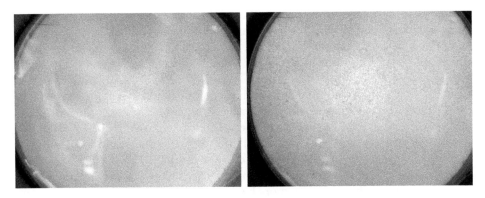

Figure 2.8 A large opening (right) will admit more light into the camera obscura, brightening the image, but will also lead to a much blurrier image than we will get with a small opening (left). Photos by the author.

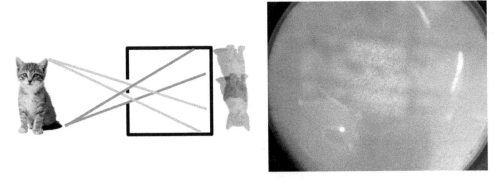

Figure 2.9 Adding two apertures to your camera leads to a doubled image. This means that your total projection of the scene is really two copies of the same image overlaid on one another and shifted by a small amount. At left, you can see the geometry of how this works as light travels from an object through each of the two pinholes to the viewing screen. At right, you can see an image I took with a double-aperture pinhole camera showing off a doubled image of the building from the earlier figures. Illustration and photo by the author.

What it means is that your pinhole camera has a case of double vision. Instead of one bright image, you'll see two copies of the outside pattern of light offset from each other by a short distance. If you have a second cardboard box available, I'd encourage you to try this two-holed camera out to confirm that this is the case. This is happening because light now has *two* ways to get into the camera from a single point on the object: It can go through one hole, or it can go through the other. These two points of entry mean that light from one part of the object ends up at two places on the viewing screen. The result? A brighter image that isn't appropriately organized spatially: Light from one object or surface ends up in two different places in your eye.

Remember, we're hoping to figure out what's going on with a large pinhole – not a camera that's got two holes in it. But here's the thing about a large pinhole: a large hole is really just a whole bunch of small holes all lined up next to each other. That means that a large pinhole gives light from one part of the object lots of different ways to get to the viewing screen. The consequence of this is not a double image, but many, many copies of the image all projected on top one another, and each one in a slightly different place. This displacement of the light coming from each part of the object across the screen is the source of the blurriness you observe when you make your pinhole larger in the model eye.

What can we do about this? Your own eye doesn't appear to have this problem, after all. When your pupil changes size, you don't experience dramatic changes in image blur, so there must be some principle of image formation we're missing. What would be nice is if we had some means of lining up the different copies of the image that are displaced across the surface of the retina. That is, having more light enter the eye is good, but we also want to ensure that light from one part of the object only gets to one part of the retina.

But wait! *This is something we know how to do.* Remember the behaviors of light that we've already discussed: Light can be *reflected, refracted,* and *diffracted.* Of these, reflection and refraction involve changing the direction of light via lawful relationships, which sounds like what we'd like to make happen here. We'd like to be able to change the direction of the light inside the camera so that the images from the two pinholes (or the rays passing through a large opening) aren't misaligned anymore.

If we start with our two-hole pinhole camera, we could change the direction of the light at each pinhole with a small prism (which could be made of glass or acrylic) placed right in front of each opening so that the light bends at the right angle to line up with the image coming through the other opening. Specifically, we could use Snell's Law to work out the right angles for the prism's sides so that we bend the light by just the right amount to line up our two images. In Figure 2.10, I've got a little schematic of what that might look like.

Your pinhole camera with a large pupil doesn't have a two-pinhole problem, however, but a large pinhole problem. But if a large pinhole is the same as a lot of little pinholes, what we need to do is make sure that the light that comes in through all of those little openings gets refracted by just the right amount to line up with the other light rays coming from the same part of the object. That's not a problem; we can just put a prism in front of each imaginary small pinhole with a slightly different angle to bend the light that passes through that point by the right amount. Specifically, the further away the pinhole

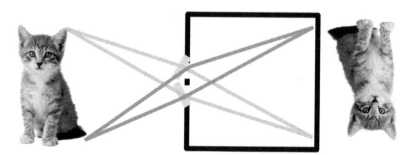

Figure 2.10 If we only had two pinholes to think about, two prisms would allow us to redirect light that passes through each hole so that our two copies of the image would be aligned with one another and not blurry. Illustration by the author.

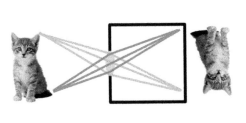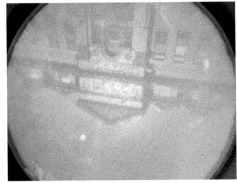

Figure 2.11 One large hole is really like having a lot of small holes next to one another. This means that we can use a smoothly curved lens to act like many prisms with different orientations to align the light that passes through each part of the opening (left). The result should be an image that is bright and clear. Illustration and photo by the author.

is from the center of the camera, the further the prism's faces will have to be tilted away from vertical. Light coming in at the center doesn't need to be bent at all, so we'll just put a vertical prism there, for example, but as we move away from the center, we'll need prism faces with more tilt to get the light to bend the correct amount. If we keep poking holes and keep putting these prisms in front of them, you would see that after a while we poke enough holes to have one big opening, and also that we've put down enough prisms with different tilts to have something new: A *lens* (Figure 2.11).

At last, let's return to your altered pinhole camera with an opening that is too large for a clear image. If you attach a biconvex lens to the front of the camera (covering the pinhole), you should be able to see a dramatic change in the image on the viewing screen. The lens should serve to refract incoming light by the right amount so that the multiple copies of the image that we're admitting into the pinhole chamber are now much better aligned. The result, once you look at your real-world scene again, should be an image that is much brighter and much clearer.

We've added something to our model eyeball, so what does this have to do with the human eye? The acrylic lens that you placed in front of your camera aperture is analogous to the cornea and/or the crystalline lens of the human eye. Both of these structures refract incoming light in the same manner as your acrylic lens to help manage the same tradeoff between image brightness and image blur. The cornea has a spherical shape that is essentially fixed, which means that it's focal length is also fixed – it will always focus light at one point in the eye. The crystalline lens can do a little more work because it can change shape, thus changing how much light rays will continue to bend as they pass through it. Together, these two structures make it possible to organize incoming light across a range of viewing distances so that you end up with relatively clear images on the retina. There are limits to this, of course. If you hold something close enough to your eye, for example, you should find that there is a distance at which you simply cannot bring the object into focus no matter what you do. This *near point* is partly the result of a constraint on how much your crystalline lens can change shape to refract incoming light by the necessary amount.

Overall, these observations highlight how the pupil, the cornea and crystalline lens, and the sclera each contribute to image formation. The variable size of the pupil allows more or less light to enter the eye, which contributes to a brighter or dimmer image as we could observe with our model pinhole. A wider aperture introduces the problem of a blurry image, however, which requires correction using a lens. With a lens that is appropriate to the size of our eye (specifically the length of our eye), we can see how an inverted image that is clear and bright can be projected onto the retinal surface.

Correcting Myopia in a Pinhole Camera

In our previous set of observations, we saw how image quality on the retina depended on the pupil, the cornea, and the crystalline lens, each represented in our pinhole camera by one of the physical parts of the model. We ignored an essential piece of the pinhole camera that does turn out to make it's own contribution to image formation however: The sclera! In our model, the sclera is represented by the cardboard box that we used to house the other elements, and we took a property of that box for granted that we're going to examine here. If you suffer from either near-sightedness or far-sightedness, you should get some insights into the nature of your vision after we're done, too. These common conditions are consequences of a mismatch between the geometry of the eye and the refractive tissues (the cornea and the crystalline lens) that contribute to the formation of sharp images projected on the retina. In this exercise, we'll use a series of different pinhole cameras to explore the nature of myopia (near-sightedness) in particular and see how it can be corrected with eyeglasses (Figure 2.12).

Things you will need:

- Some cardboard cylinders of different sizes – I've found that the good folks at Pringles make tubes in a convenient variety of sizes, but as long as you have boxes, tubes, or some other cardboard enclosure of different lengths this will work.

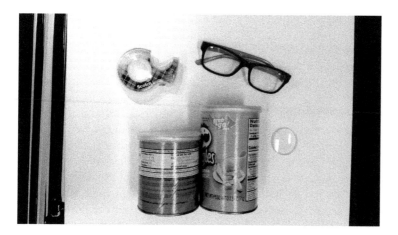

Figure 2.12 Pringles tubes are a convenient way to make pinhole cameras with different lengths so that we can observe how near-sightedness and far-sightedness work. Photo by the author.

- A small amount of tracing paper. You only need a piece big enough to cover the opening of your cylinder or tube.
- A biconvex lens with a focal length close to the box size.
- Some reading glasses. I'd recommend getting a multi-pack covering a range of positive and negative diopter values.

Building a Pringles Pinhole Camera

Our first step is to build a basic pinhole camera out of the shortest tube that we have on hand. If you are indeed using a Pringles tube (or similar product), there are just two main steps to complete: (1) Punch a hole in the middle of the bottom surface of the tube, and (2) Cut a circle of tracing paper that will fit just inside the tube's plastic lid. If the tube(s) you are using do not have a lid, I'd recommend using some type of cling film to help secure your tracing paper across one end of the tube (Figure 2.13).

Once you have done that, you should be able to see some images projected on the viewing screen by pointing the opening at a bright scene or a nearby light source. To make those images much brighter and sharper, attach your lens in front of the hole you punched. Hopefully, you will once again be able to see a nice projection of a real-world scene onto your tracing paper. Now, repeat these steps for your tube that is slightly longer, and you should notice a problem. While the image in your short tube was probably clear, the image in the longer tube should be blurrier. But why? We have all the pieces that we said were crucial to good image formation, but something still isn't working the way that we want. Again, we need to revisit the principles of geometric optics that we learned about earlier to understand the nature of this problem and how we might address it by modifying our camera (Figure 2.14).

The problem here is that the different copies of the image entering your pinhole from different directions are being aligned by the lens we have installed, but that alignment is happening *in front* of your viewing screen rather than on it. This is happening because of a natural consequence of Snell's Law and the lens that we've installed in this pinhole

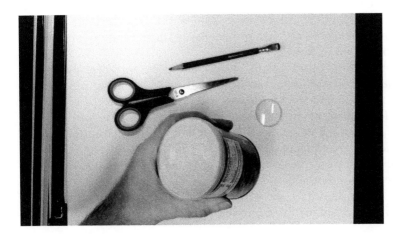

Figure 2.13 We can make a simple pinhole camera out of each tube by repeating our steps from the previous exercise. Photo by the author.

Original Tube (matched to lens)   Longer Tube

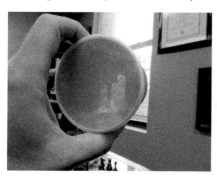 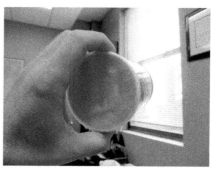

Figure 2.14 While a short tube will likely yield a clear image once the lens is installed (left), a longer tube will look blurrier with the same lens (right). This is the same problem facing myopic individuals: Their eyes are ovoid shaped rather than spherical. Photo by the author.

camera. Remember that we learned that both concave and convex lenses had a property called the *focal length*. This referred to the distance at which incoming light rays that were perpendicular to the lens axis converged at a common point that was opposite the incoming light for a convex lens and on the same side as the incoming light for a concave lens. The property of the sclera (and the pinhole camera body) that we haven't been very careful about so far is its size relative to the lens that we use to converge incoming light rays on the retina. In an ideal world, the length of the sclera should match the focal length of the lens that we position at the front of the eye. This would ensure that the incoming light rays are organized the way that we want right on the surface of the retina.

The problem that we're seeing once we switch to the longer tube is a consequence of a mismatch between these two lengths. The lens that we're using is still converging the light rays the same way that it was in the first camera, but now the retina is further away from the lens than it was in the original model. This means that the rays of light that we'd like to have meet up do converge, but then they diverge again before they arrive at the tracing paper. This is exactly the problem people with myopia have: Their eye is too long relative to the shape of their cornea and its focal length.

What can we do about this? The way we fix myopia for people with near-sightedness is simple: We have them wear another lens in front of their own cornea, which bends incoming light by the right amount so that the subsequent bending that the cornea and lens do will lead to a focused image on the retina. If you wear glasses or contacts, your prescription is a description of the shape this additional lens needs to be so that light is bent by the proper amount. Try correcting the image in your longer tube by holding up either your own glasses if you wear them or the different pairs of reading glasses in front of the lens until you see an improvement in the image. You ought to be able to find one that does a reasonable job tidying things up. Once you do, make a note of what kind of lens it is (e.g., +2, –1.5) and experiment with shorter or longer tubes if you have them on hand (Figure 2.15).

Longer tube (again)   Longer Tube w/eyeglasses

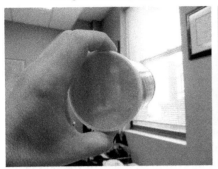 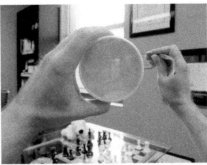

Figure 2.15 Giving our longer tube some glasses (in this case, my own prescription) improves our image quality. Photo by the author.

This should give you a basic sense of how understanding the optics of refraction helps us compensate for variation in the shape of the eye and the cornea that would otherwise compromise image formation and subjective image quality. These principles can get you a long way in terms of thinking through other common optical conditions, too. If near-sightedness is the result of a sclera that is too long, you probably won't be surprised to hear that far-sightedness is the result of a sclera that is too short, for example. To go just a little further, you can also probably start to imagine what we'd like light to do so that we correct for a far-sighted sclera, and link this to lens shape, by remembering your geometric optics principles. Another optical condition, astigmatism, results from differential curvature of the cornea along the horizontal and vertical axes. That is, instead of having a cornea that's shaped like a cap you might cut off from a sphere, an astigmatic cornea is shaped more like an American football or a rugby ball. The consequence is that light is being refracted differently depending on which way it enters the eye, but again, we can try to correct this with modifications to a corrective lens that we introduce into the overall optical configuration. In all of these cases, the key idea to keep in mind is that we have quantitative tools to make sure light is bent by appropriate amounts to accommodate different properties of the eye itself.

Observing the Inverted Retinal Image

In the two previous pinhole camera exercises, you were able to observe that the image projected onto the back of the camera was an upside-down and reversed version of the actual scene you were pointing the camera towards. Is the image on your own retina also inverted? The possibility that it might be seemed to a number of experimental philosophers like something that needed to be explained (Wade, 1998), with some of them going so far as to propose that the optics of the eye, to yield a focused and upright image instead of an inverted one, must be more complicated than we've presumed. The retinal image *is* inverted, though, and we can see this if we look at the eye with an ophthalmoscope or if we dissect a real eye and project images into it. In this exercise, however, we'll give you the chance to see evidence of this just by casting a shadow on your retina (Balas & McCourt, 2023).

Things you will need:

- An eye (preferably yours).
- A piece of cardstock (a 3" × 5" card or business card works well).
- A thumbtack or needle.
- A sharpened pencil.

Casting a Shadow on Your Retina with Collimated Light

To make this effect work, we need a collimated light source. This refers to light that is streaming towards us with parallel rays (not diverging as they travel) that are perpendicular to the frontal plane of the eye. If that sounds complicated, what I mean is that collimated light in this case will be traveling straight towards your eye without any of the rays being bent upwards, downwards, or off to one side or the other. Our plan is not to go find a collimated light source, but to approximate one by forcing light to stream through a small hole in our piece of cardstock. This approximation is convenient, but also means that light isn't perfectly straight after coming through the hole. The trick will be to manage how far we make the light rays travel between this pinhole and our eye.

Begin by puncturing a hole in the card with your thumbtack and widen it just a bit by pushing the tip of your pencil partway into it. The hole should be just about 2mm wide. That specific number isn't particularly important, but you don't want this opening to be too large. If it is, incoming light will be imperfectly collimated even after passing straight through it.

The tricky part of achieving the effect that we're looking for is making sure we align all of the elements that we need appropriately to give us what we're looking for. Before you go look at the diagram in Figure 2.16, here's the intuition for what we're trying to do: We want light to stream through this pinhole and towards our eye like a tiny spotlight, and we also want to put the tip of our pencil in the way of this spotlight so we cast the shadow of the pencil on our retina. With that in mind, take a look at Figure 2.16 to see what you need to do – getting these distances at least approximately right really matters! Notice in particular that the pencil is quite close to your face, while the card should be further away.

If you've got everything set up correctly, you should be able to see two things: (1) The pencil tip itself should be visible to you and it should look quite blurry given how close it is to your eye. It looks blurry because it is too close for your crystalline lens to flex enough to adequately refract the divergent light coming from it towards your eye; (2) The shadow of the pencil tip should be visible, but it should be on the opposite side of your "spotlight!" If you move the pencil tip slowly upwards, you should see the shadow move downwards (Figure 2.17).

Why Is This Happening?

Figure 2.18 illustrates what is happening to the light coming from various parts of this small scene. The diverging light from the pencil is focused by the cornea and ultimately refracts onto the retina as illustrated. Hopefully it's not too difficult to think through why the light should take the path that I've drawn in Figure 2.18 based on your prior observations of refraction. The collimated light from the pinhole, however, refracts as shown, and the pencil's shadow is an interruption of that light that doesn't "switch sides" on the way in (Figure 2.18).

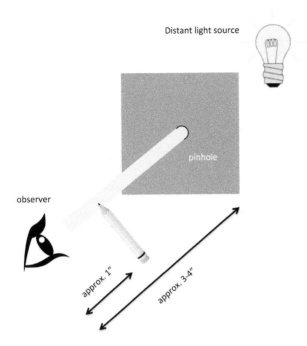

Figure 2.16 This arrangement of the card, the pencil, a light source, and your eye is critical to observing this effect. Be careful with the distances! Figure from Balas and McCourt (2023).

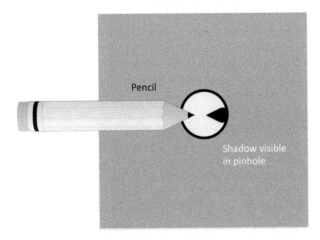

Figure 2.17 If you've got our optical set-up correct, you should be able to see the actual tip of your pencil and the reversed shadow of the pencil intruding on the other side of the light! Figure from Balas and McCourt (2023).

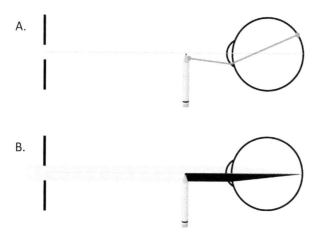

Figure 2.18 A schematic diagram of what light rays and shadows are doing in this set-up to yield the phenomenon above. Figure from Balas and McCourt (2023).

This neat little effect gives you a chance to see that your own optical set-up in the eye really does yield an inverted image. The shadow looks reversed to you because it's the only thing that isn't optically reversed in this configuration! That means that the image of the pencil tip is reversed, but that your visual system delivers a subjective experience of the world that is nonetheless upright and in the original left-right arrangement.

As I mentioned above, some early perspectives on image formation included various explanations of how the inverted image might be optically flipped to ensure that we didn't have to worry about how we see an upright world. I won't talk through these ideas here, but thinking through what kinds of reflections or refractions you might add to the optics of the eye to achieve an upright image on the retina is an interesting problem that requires careful use of the lawful behaviors of light that we observed earlier. Our own visual system doesn't need these complicated mechanisms, however, yielding an upright experience of the world regardless of the inverted image at the back of the eye. How does it do this? I think that the simplest answer is that the orientation of the image on the back of the eye is, ultimately, sort of arbitrary: What matters is how the next stages of vision unfold. How do the photoreceptors in the retina send information onto the next cells in the visual system? If you were really worried about the spatial arrangement of the image, you could easily imagine that there is just some sort of crossing-over at later stages so that we manage the orientation of the image appropriately. A more abstract way to think about the issue is to consider that mapping physical properties like the position of the photoreceptors on the retina to perceptual outcomes like your experience of the world may be much more complex than simply putting signals in place perceptually in exactly the same arrangement they were measured in physically.

This latter idea is an important one because it is a precursor to one of the most important properties of your visual system: The measurements you start with are the beginning of your perceptual experience, not the end! Visual processing involves a great deal of work to go beyond the raw measurement of light to deliver a subjective experience to you that supports understanding your visual world and how to plan action within it. Seeing an upright image after obtaining an inverted retinal projection of the world shares something with many of the other phenomena we will encounter in that we start with some measurement and use this to infer or guess something about the visual world. We still have a number of different aspects of measurement to consider, but all of these will ultimately be the basis for taking steps beyond the raw data to get to something richer.

References

Balas, B., & McCourt, M. (2023). Casting shadows on the eye to reveal the inverted retinal image. *Visual Cognition*.

Cabe, P. A. (2003). A ping-pong ball camera obscura. *Perception, 32*(7), 895–896. https://doi.org /10.1068/p5042

Cabe, P. A. (2018). Multi-Image pinhole viewer using a biscuit. *Perception, 47*(1), 112–114. https://doi.org/10.1177/0301006617739756

Wade, N. J. (1998). *A natural history of vision.* MIT Press.

Wade, N. J., & Finger, S. (2001). The eye as an optical instrument: From camera obscura to Helmholtz's perspective. *Perception, 30*(10), 1157–1177. https://doi.org/10.1068/p3210

Young, M. (1971). Pinhole optics. *Applied Optics, 10*(12), 2763–2767. https://doi.org/10.1364 /AO.10.002763

3 Measuring Light with the Retina

In our previous chapter, we described the interaction of the cornea, crystalline lens, pupil, and sclera to facilitate the formation of a clear and bright image at the back of the eye. The pinhole camera that we built to examine image formation included only a crude model retina (a sheet of tracing paper) that served only to give us a view of the image we could form with the other elements of the camera. The human eye has a much more elaborate structure called the *retina* (Figure 3.1) where images are formed at the back of the eye. The retina includes special cells called *photoreceptors* that carry out a process called *transduction*, which refers to the transformation of light into the electrical signals cells in the nervous system use to process information. There are two main varieties of photoreceptor cells, the rods and cones, that differ from one another according to their sensitivity to varying wavelengths of light. That difference in how these photoreceptors absorb light of different wavelengths supports our ability to estimate the wavelength content of incoming

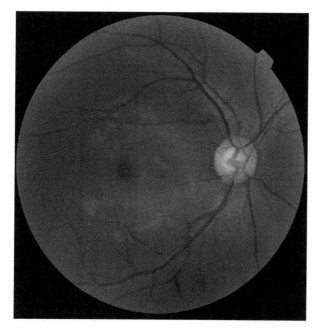

Figure 3.1 A view of the human retina through an ophthalmoscope. Image credit: Ske., CC BY-SA 3.0 <http://creativecommons.org/licenses/by-sa/3.0/>, via Wikimedia Commons.

DOI: 10.4324/9781032691169-4

light. Our goal in this chapter is to explore several different aspects of the retina's structure and its function. The **Sunprint Photography** exercises give you a chance to see what wavelength selectivity is like in a model photopigment called a cyanotype. By working with a photopigment you can easily expose to different kinds of light, you can build intuitions for how the rods and cones differ from one another in terms of how they respond to incoming light. A crucial difference between our sunprint paper and the real retina however, is that the real retina is not uniform across its surface. The **Retinal Blind Spot** exercise reveals the extent of a profound retinal inhomogeneity: The complete absence of photoreceptors from a region in each eye. Finally, the retina is positioned behind a layer of capillaries which are generally not visible during normal situations. The **Draw Your Own Retina** exercise makes them visible however, in a way that reveals some of the structural architecture of the eye and the retina itself.

Draw Your Own Retinal Vasculature

The pinhole cameras that we worked with in the previous chapter were a much-simplified model of the human eye that helped us understand some important aspects of image formation. Your own eye includes a number of features that we didn't incorporate into our paper models, of course, some of which we can observe to gain additional insight into how the next steps in seeing work. Here, we are going to take advantage of an entoptic phenomenon to draw the retinal vasculature in your own eye.

An *entoptic phenomenon* refers to some kind of visual experience that originates within the eye rather than coming from the external visual environment. If you've ever seen "floaters" in your field of view, or small, sparkling white dots at the edges of your vision when you look up at a clear blue sky, both of these are examples of entopic phenomena. In the former case (floaters) what you are seeing are the shadows cast by coagulated pieces of the vitreous humor that are floating inside the eye, and, in the latter case, you are seeing the shadows of blood cells making their way through the small blood vessels that are arranged between the retina and the front of the eye.

Yes, you heard that right: Small blood vessels lie between the retina and the light that's coming into the eye. This may seem to you like a strange way for an eye to be put together. Don't those blood vessels block some of the incoming light and make it harder to see things? Thankfully, we don't usually see these vessels due to a number of optical factors. What we're going to do in this exercise though is make them visible using a simple technique so that you can both see them and try to draw what they look like to you. By observing the layout of these blood vessels, we should also be able to learn something important about the architecture of the retina that presages some important concepts we will elaborate on more in subsequent chapters.

Things you will need:

- An eyeball (yours).
- A small flashlight.
- Things to draw with.

Casting Shadows on Your Retina

To see these blood vessels, we'll use a flashlight to cast their shadows on the retina. This isn't quite as reliable as using a slit-lamp (like you might find at your eye doctor's office), which can give you particularly nice views of this vasculature (Bradley et al., 1998), but it should get the job done. What we should get from following these instructions is a fleeting glimpse of the branching network of these vessels covering your whole visual field, probably in a sort of purply-yellow haze. This is hard to articulate but quite vivid once you get the technique down. One thing that we need to be clear about before we start, however, is this: We are not talking about the small blood vessels that you can see on the surface of your sclera if you look at your eye in a normal mirror. Instead, we are going to use an optical trick to help you see the blood vessels that are *in* your eye rather than *on* your eye. Your experience of seeing them is going to be quite different than what it's like to look at your eye in a mirror, so be prepared for a different kind of visual phenomenon.

To get this to work, you're going to try and shine light obliquely into your pupil. First, a cautionary note: Do NOT use a laser pointer or other high-power light source for this effect! You should use an ordinary flashlight to ensure that you don't damage your eye with light that is too intense. Next, I'm going to suggest that you head for a relatively dark room to limit the ambient light getting into your eye through other means. Finally, I've found that the best way to do this is to close one eye, turn the open eye towards your nose (if it's your left eye, look right), and then jiggle the flashlight beam towards the opposite corner of that eye (if it's your left eye, looking right, shine the light into the left side of that eye). What you should see as you jiggle the light is a sudden pattern of spidery branches filling up your visual field. The visibility of these branches (which are indeed the blood vessels we are interested in!) will depend a lot on moving the light, so keep jiggling your light source while trying to pay attention to the layout of the branches across your field of view. Try to draw what you see as best as you can, but also give yourself breaks as needed so you don't get overwhelmed by shining a flashlight into your eye (Figure 3.2).

The Retinal Vasculature and the Blind Spot

This can be pretty tough to do if I'm being honest, as your view of these blood vessels tends to be only very brief. Still, if you stick with it, you will likely at least be able to see

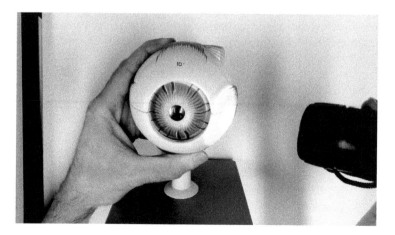

Figure 3.2 Shining light obliquely onto the retina through the white part of the eye should lead to cast shadows from the blood vessels we want to observe on the retina. Photo by the author.

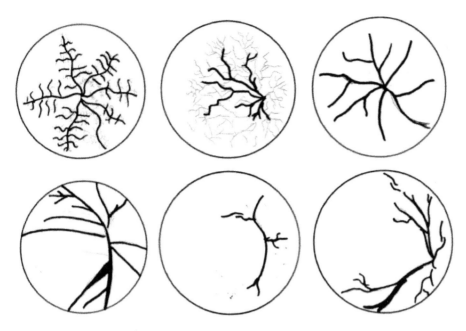

Figure 3.3 Examples of students' drawings of their retinal vasculature. Note the convergence of the lines on the right side of the image. Photo by the author.

something. In particular, one feature a lot of students are able to see is a very large X-shape off to the outer side of their visual field. In Figure 3.3 you can see some student depictions from my classes that include this feature to varying degrees. You can also go take a look at the image of a retina viewed with an ophthalmoscope at the beginning of this chapter, where these large crossing contours are very conspicuous at the right side of the image (Figure 3.1).

If you're able to look for these vessels in both your left and right eye, you should find that this X-like structure is evident in both eyes, but on opposite sides: It should be off to the right side in your right eye and off to the left side in your left eye. You should also find that if you compare drawings with other people, there ought to be good consistency about the shape and position of these largest vessels. This consistency is a hint that this is an important structural feature of the eye that's worthy of further attention and explanation.

To offer that explanation (which we'll build on in the next section), the convergence of blood vessels at this point is indeed an important structural inhomogeneity within the eye. The center of this X is the place where blood vessels and the axons of cells in our retina exit the eye. The eye can't be a self-contained and complete organ after all, so there has to be some kind of connection between the eye and the rest of the nervous system. The catch is that because of the way our eye is structured, this exit portal ends up taking some space on the retina, which is where we're trying to record incoming light! This means that there ought to be a part of our visual field in each eye that is completely blind to incoming light because there are no cells there to measure it. This "blind spot" is both an interesting structural and functional fact in its own right, but also ends up revealing some important ways in which your visual system treats raw sense data as a starting point for visual experience that is elaborated upon through various kinds of guesswork and inference. We'll continue by playing with this blind spot further to see what it's like to see without actually seeing anything.

Finding Your Retinal Blind Spot.

Now that we've looked at your retina vasculature and identified that there is a blind spot in each of your two retinae where blood vessels and axons exit the eye to interface with the rest of the nervous system, let's examine some features of this no-man's-land where your photoreceptors don't measure anything. A first observation, or perhaps simply an intuition, about your visual experience with regard to this blind spot is that you probably don't feel much like you have one as you look around the world. If there really is a spot on each of your retinae where you aren't able to measure any light, why shouldn't you see some sort of hole in your visual field?

This hypothesis about what the consequences of the blind spot ought to be on your visual experience depends in part on an idea that we should make explicit now because we will need it later: The idea of a *receptive field* for cells in your visual system that measure light. Although we haven't actually said much about discrete cells in your retina or in other parts of your visual system yet, we will do so soon, and this term is an important property to keep in mind with regard to those cells and how they process light. The term receptive field refers to the portion of the visual field where light may influence the response of a cell. A simple way to think about this is to imagine that each part of the retina, for example, only sees the visual world through a small window. Light that is beyond the borders of that window is not measured by that part of the retina, but the entire visual field is accounted for by different parts of the retinal surface. To return to our initial impressions of the blind spot, what we're really saying is that it seems like the empty portion of the retina might imply that there is a corresponding portion of the visual world that doesn't have a "window" which makes it a little strange that we still experience a visual world with no gaps in it.

What we will observe in this exercise is that your visual experience does in fact have holes in it, but your visual system also apparently has some interesting ways to get around this. Our goal is to give yourself a chance to experience this gap in your measurement of light at the retina, observe some properties of the blind spot in terms of the visual environment, and finally to test the limits of your visual system's mechanisms for "filling in" your visual experience (Anstis, 2010).

Things you will need:

- An eyeball (yours).
- A picture of some dots and a dashed vertical line (see supplementary material).

1) With your left eye closed, hold the first page so that the dashed line is to the left and the circles are on the right side of the page.
2) Look with your right eye only at the top of the dashed line. The smallest black circle should be off to the right of where you are looking.
3) Move the paper slowly forwards or backwards until that smallest circle vanishes completely.
4) Repeat by looking a little further down on the dashed line, and see if you can get each of the bigger circles to vanish completely.

The first thing to take note of as you carry out these steps is that you should be able to get at least the smallest circle to vanish completely! This is noteworthy because it means that the blind spot really is blind when tested the right way. The critical step, of course, was restricting your visual experience to what you could see with one eye. This difference between vision with one eye (or *monocular vision*) and vision with two eyes (or *binocular vision*) suggests a straightforward solution to our earlier conundrum: Your visual experience does not include "holes" corresponding to the blind spots in the two retinae because your visual system must be able to rely on the information from one eye to provide the missing measurements that correspond to the blind spot in the other eye. Viewing these dots monocularly removes the ability to do so, making it possible to see (or rather, to not see) your blind spot.

The graded size of the different test circles also gives us a chance to estimate how big the blind spot is in terms of the amount of the visual field that is missing. Now seems like a good time to introduce a term of art that refers to the way we tend to talk about spatial extent in circumstances like this, so let's take a moment to discuss *visual angle* and how to calculate it. Briefly, rather than measure the amount of area taken up by something in our visual field using units like inches or centimeters, we usually describe size in terms of an angle. This may seem a little cumbersome at first, but it turns out to be the most straightforward thing to do. In Figure 3.4, you can see how we can calculate visual angle based on the distance between ourselves and an object and the actual size of that object. If I'm being honest about it, however, I often use an actual rule of thumb to estimate the visual angle subtended by different objects: Your thumb extended at arm's length is about

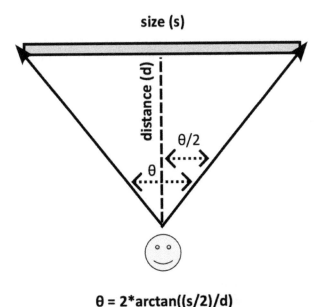

$$\theta = 2*arctan((s/2)/d)$$

Figure 3.4 We calculate visual angle as a way to talk about amount of space something takes up in our visual field. This diagram includes the formula for visual angle at right as a function of the size of the object and viewing distance while also depicting where that formula comes from. Illustration by the author.

as wide as 2 degrees of visual angle, which means you can quickly estimate image area by using your thumb as a ruler. If you feel ambitious, you might try measuring the size of your blind spot by estimating the visual angle taken up by the smallest disc that you can't make completely vanish. You can also try closing an eye and moving your thumb around at arm's length to test the boundaries of the blind spot while you measure. Either method should give an estimate of about 5–6 degrees wide, and about 7–8 degrees tall (Figure 3.4).

Now to turn our attention to a potentially more interesting property of the blind spot, or rather, your visual experience inside the blind spot. Note that, when each circle disappears, the white background of the paper is filled in to the empty space. You don't see an empty black hole, but instead see a continuous field of white. This is interesting because it suggests that even in the absence of the information from your other eye, your visual system can do something to offer you a subjective experience of the world that doesn't have a hole in it. But how much can it offer? Take a look at the second sheet of images in the supplementary material to see if your visual system can complete textures, contours, or even complicated shapes when parts of these forms fall into the blind spot. You can also take a look at Figure 3.5 to get the same kind of effect: Look at the black cross with your right eye and move until the red dot is in your blind spot. Do you still see the brick-like texture? Most people find that while simple textures and contours are completed easily, more complex shapes are not.

This is another case where you might find it interesting to test some of the limits of blind spot perception: For example, are there texture patterns that your visual system fills in more effectively than others? What happens when contours that lie on either side of the blind spot are more or less similar to one another in terms of their angle, their color, or their size? Finally, a very complex object doesn't appear to be filled in very well, but can you make an object simple enough that you do get something convincing? Whether you probe the limits of this phenomenon or not, this is another excellent example of your visual system doing something more than simply recording light and telling you about the raw measurement. The filling-in or completion of missing information in the blind spot under monocular viewing conditions is a form of guesswork, or inference. Your visual system is going beyond the data that it has to make estimates of what is really out there, and your experience of the visual world is the product of that estimation. We'll need this idea again very soon, so don't forget that this is a key aspect of visual perception!

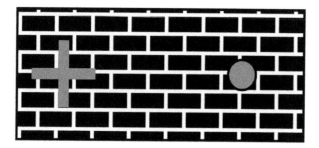

Figure 3.5 A quick demonstration of filling-in of texture inside the blind spot. Even when the red dot disappears under monocular viewing, the brick texture should appear uniform. Illustration by the author.

Sunprint Photography – Investigating Wavelength Selectivity with a Model Retina

Now we're on to a serious step: After images are formed in the eye, the next step is the transduction of that light by the retina to produce a signal that the nervous system can use for subsequent processing. The retina achieves this with special cells called photoreceptors that absorb light and produce an electrical response. That response serves as the starting point for our visual system to confer a visual experience, so understanding how the properties of light affect the responses of these cells is very important.

Different photoreceptors in the retina absorb light differently as a function of wavelength, which is the basis for our ability to distinguish lights based on the wavelength ingredients that they are made up of and thus experience color. In this exercise, we'll explore what it means for a photosensitive material to absorb light as a function of wavelength by working with sunprint paper. We'll also examine how the intensity of incoming light and the wavelength of incoming light both affect the response that we get from a photopigment. The fact that both of these properties of light influence the strength of the signal that a photopigment generates has important consequences for how our visual system uses photoreceptor responses to infer something about the wavelength content of incoming light (Figure 3.6).

Things you will need:

- Sunprint paper (many vendors for this, any are probably fine).
- Laser pointers (red, green, and blue).
- An ultraviolet flashlight – 395nm is easiest to find, but if you can go shorter wavelength, go for it.
- An aluminum baking tray.
- An index card with a large hole cut out of it.
- A neutral density filter (I recommend a gray/clear binder divider).
- A stopwatch of some kind (I use an hourglass solely for style points).

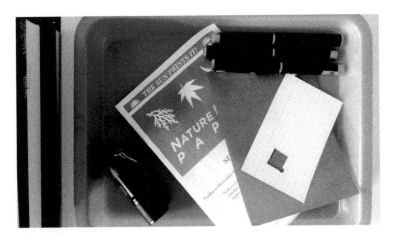

Figure 3.6 We can make cyanotypes with sunprint paper, water, some different light sources (red, green, and blue laser pointers and a UV light) and an occluding window. Photo by the author.

How Does Photopigment Response Vary with Light Intensity?

Our first step is to examine how the intensity of a light source affects the response of a photopigment. We'll do this using a light with a fixed intensity (the sun) but varying the amount of light our photopigment absorbs by exposing it to sunlight for different amounts of time. To do this in a controlled way, cut a small hole out of an opaque piece of paper so that you can leave only a small part of the sunprint paper open to the sun. Go outside and expose this part of the sunprint film to sunlight for ~15 seconds, then move your occluding card around so you can expose a different part of the film to the light for ~30 seconds, and finally do this again for an exposure time of ~60 seconds or so. You may be able to see the paper start to bleach while you're counting down the seconds, but don't worry if you can't. Once you're done with your three exposures, submerge the whole paper in water (check the instructions on your particular brand of sunprint paper to confirm how to do this). This will stop the photopigment reaction and fix the responses to the different amounts of light. You should be able to see some darkened marks on the paper that correspond to your different exposures (Figure 3.7).

If you look a little closer, you should be able to see that the different squares are darker in tone as the exposure time increased: Your 60-second exposure ought to look much darker than your 15-second exposure, for example, and the 30-second exposure should be somewhere in between. More intense light thus led to a larger response from this photopigment, in the form of a more substantial change in the pigment itself as time increased.

To get you thinking about what kind of information we'd like to be able to get from our visual system based on the way different cells respond to light, consider whether or not you'd be able to run this process in reverse. That is, given what you know now, what if I handed you a fully developed piece of sunprint paper and asked you to look at the marks to determine how long the film had been exposed to light? It's tempting to think that this wouldn't be so hard: With some careful measurement of precisely how dark each exposed portion of the paper is and a standard of some kind to compare it to, it certainly seems like we might be able to get good estimates of exposure time based on the appearance of the

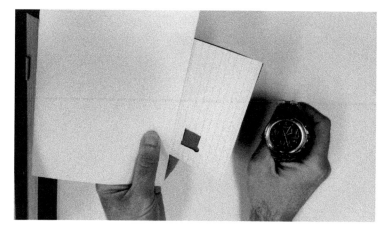

Figure 3.7 Use the occluder to control what part of the sunprint paper you expose to different lights for varying amounts of time. Photo by the author.

sunprint. This is potentially a useful trick because it means we can start with a measurement by the photoreceptors and work backwards to an estimate of what was actually happening in the environment that gave rise to the values we obtained. That kind of estimation is fundamental to how we end up with an experience of the visual world based on what the cells in our visual system are doing to respond to it.

The situation is more complicated than that, however, and to see why I'd like you to go back outside with more sunprint paper and the neutral density filter listed above. This can be something as simple as a bit of grayish plastic that you can mostly see through, or even a dusty bit of cling film. Whatever material you're using, repeat the steps described previously with the same three exposure times (15, 30, and 60 seconds) but with the neutral density filter covering the sunprint paper. The fact that this filter is translucent means that light is getting through, but how does it affect your results? After you develop your sunprint paper, you should find that the same three exposure times led to marks on the paper that were much less vivid. This may seem like an elementary point, but it's a very important one: By limiting how much light actually got to the paper (varying the intensity of the light), we changed the relationship between exposure time and the darkness of the mark on the paper. This means that we have a much more difficult inference problem than we thought – the darkness of the developed sunprint film depends on two variables (exposure time and light-source intensity), but we only get one number out of the developed paper. This kind of situation is a classic example of an *underconstrained problem*, and this is only the beginning of our encounters with this conundrum. For now, I just want you to remember that we'd love to be able to use our measurements to make inferences about the environment, but in this case, we have limited information to base this guesswork on. As we'll see in a moment, the situation is even more complicated than this.

How Does Photopigment Response Vary with Wavelength?

Next, we'll investigate how our photopigment responds to lights with roughly the same intensity but different wavelengths. We'll achieve this by using laser pointers to illuminate the sunprint paper instead of the sun. The convenient thing about these light sources is that while different colors of laser pointer tend to have fairly consistent intensity, we've already seen that they differ in wavelength. A red laser pointer usually emits light with a wavelength of about 650nm, a green laser pointer usually has a wavelength of about 530nm, and a blue laser point usually has a wavelength of about 415nm. If you recall what we saw when we observed laser light after it passed through a diffraction grating, it's also the case that these are very narrow-band light sources: Rather than a richer spectrum of light, they will usually have a very limited set of wavelengths. This makes them a great test of the *wavelength selectivity* of our photopigment: How does the response of the paper depend on wavelength?

For this part of the exercise, go indoors so that your paper is not exposed to sunlight and shine each of your three laser pointers on a different part of some sunprint paper for the same amount of time (I'd recommend about 15–20 seconds). Again, you may see some bleaching as the lights are being shined onto the paper, but submerge the whole paper in water once you've collected all three lights to ensure that you get your best chance to see how the paper changed in response to each light source (Figure 3.8).

In this case, you should be able to see that while the red and green laser probably didn't do much to change the way that the paper looked, the blue laser likely yielded a very dark

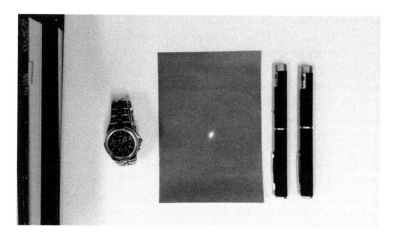

Figure 3.8 Indoors, try exposing the sunprint paper to each of the different laser pointer colors and a UV light if you have one available. Photo by the author.

dot. This tells us that this material doesn't just soak up all kinds of light, but is *selective* for wavelength. Neither red nor green light is absorbed well, but short-wavelength blue light is absorbed readily. If you have one available to you, you can try shining a UV light on the paper to see what it does, too. These light sources have an even shorter wavelength than your blue laser pointer, usually in the neighborhood of 350nm or so. If you're able to try this out, you should find that even though you can't see this light very well at all, the sunprint paper ought to change very rapidly. This tells us that short wavelengths are preferentially absorbed by this particular photopigment (Figure 3.9).

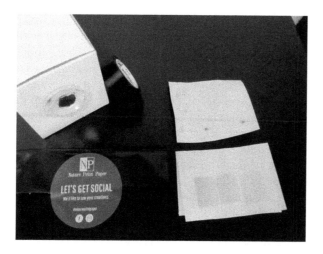

Figure 3.9 Varying the exposure time and the wavelength of incoming light should dramatically affect the darkness of the developed print. Photo by the author.

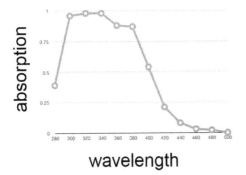

Figure 3.10 The absorption spectrum of typical sunprint paper. Short-wavelength light produces a large response, but light with a wavelength much longer than about 400nm does very little to change the paper's appearance. Illustration by the author.

Let's return to the question I posed after our first set of observations: Could we use the mark on the sunprint paper to inform some guesses about the conditions in the environment that led to this response? If we were just thinking about wavelength, we might start out feeling optimistic about this problem. Again, we'd need some kind of standard to compare the marks on our sunprint paper to, but with something like that in hand we might be able to precisely measure the response on the paper and use that to guess what wavelength the paper had been exposed to. In fact, something like this standard already exists in the form of what we call the absorption spectrum for our photopigment. This is a list of numbers (usually visualized via something like the graph in Figure 3.10) that tells us how readily the photopigment we're considering absorbs the different wavelengths of light, which is directly linked to the response that we observe on the photopigment. If you take a look at the graph of typical sunprint paper's absorption spectrum, you can see that it confirms what we've already observed: Shorter wavelengths are absorbed well, but medium to long wavelengths are absorbed poorly (Figure 3.10).

But we already know this isn't the only variable that affects the response of our photopigment. Besides wavelength, we've already seen that light source intensity and exposure time both influence the response that we can measure, so our underconstrained problem is not quite difficult. We get one response from a photopigment (operationalized here via the darkness of the exposed sunprint paper), but that response was the result of three different variables in the environment. Our situation is very much like being given a single number (let's say 120) and asked to guess which three numbers we multiplied together to obtain it. Without more information, we can't arrive at a unique solution.

This may seem like a poor state of affairs, but it's time to abandon our model retina in favor of the real thing so that we can understand more about how your visual system is capable of doing some better guesswork with regard to wavelength encoding in particular. Obviously people tend to have experiences of color, so something must be happening to provide you with information about the wavelengths of light in the world around you. But how?

If we were to look closely enough at the retina itself, we could actually see the photoreceptors that serve as the sunprint film for your eye (Thibos et al., 2023). While we treated our sunprint film as a uniform material that didn't vary across its surface, looking at the retinal photoreceptors gives us a reason to rethink this assumption: The cells that we find in the human retina have different shapes to them if we look at a portion called their *outer segment*. One kind of cell will have an outer segment that's cylindrical (or rod-shaped), while the other kind of cell will have an outer segment that tapers (or is more cone-shaped). For lack of better words, let's call these cells *rods* and *cones*. The existence of two kinds of cells raises some natural questions, including where we find one kind of cell compared to the other and what the wavelength selectivity of each kind of cell might be. If we confine ourselves to what we can work out by just looking at the cells, we'll find that the rods and cones are distributed very differently across the retina. Cones are very dense in central vision (and drop off quickly as we move towards the periphery), while cones are absent from central vision and have a sort of rise-and-fall distribution as we move to the periphery. Whatever these two kinds of photoreceptor might be doing differently from one another, they are doing their job in different parts of the visual field (Figure 3.11).

But what are they doing to transduce light? To figure out the wavelength selectivity of each photopigment, we could imagine doing something similar to what you just did with the sunprint paper. We could expose the photopigment on each kind of photoreceptor to different wavelengths of light (controlling the intensity so it didn't confound our measurements), and try to measure how much the photopigment changed in response to each kind of light. This would ideally yield an absorption spectrum like the one I showed you in Figure 3.10 for

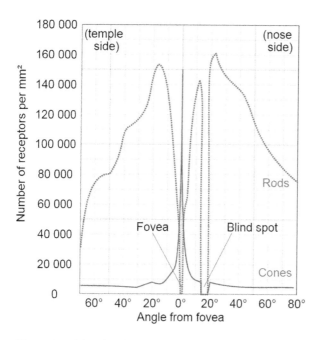

Figure 3.11 The distribution of rods and cones across the retina. Cones are densely packed into the very center of the retina, while the rods are distributed out towards the edges. Image credit: Cmglee, CC BY-SA 3.0 <https://creativecommons.org/licenses/by-sa/3.0>, via Wikimedia Commons.

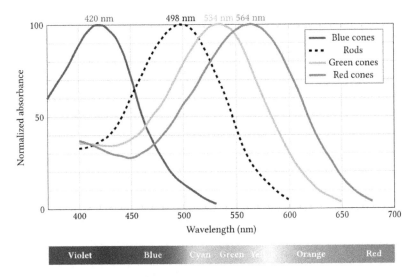

Figure 3.12 Compare the absorption functions of the three kinds of cones (depicted here in red, green, and blue curves) and the rods (in black) to the cyanotype spectrum below the graph. The fact that these cells have different absorption spectra makes it possible for our visual system to use the different responses the cones produce to the same incoming light as the basis for distinguishing light based on its wavelength and granting you the ability to see color. Public Domain image by Francois~frwiki CC BY-SA 4.0 <https:// creativecommons.org/licenses/by-sa/4.0/> via Wikimedia Commons.

the sunprint film. If we did this, how different would the rods and cones be in terms of the light they absorb more easily? The answer turns out to be that they're quite different, and the differences are even bigger than the shape of the cells' outer segments suggests. Individual rods will have an absorption spectrum that looks like the dark line in Figure 3.12, peaking in the neighborhood of 500nm and falling off fairly sharply to either side of that value. As for the cones, well, it turns out that there isn't one answer, but rather there are three different answers! Cones come in three different varieties, each with a different sensitivity to wavelength. The blue, green, and red lines in Figure 3.12 indicate the different absorption spectra we will observe from so-called short-, medium-, and long-wavelength cones, respectively. Each class of cone has a different peak sensitivity, but all three of them have a similar fall-off in sensitivity as we move away from that optimal value. Your visual system thus doesn't just have one kind of sunprint film in the eye, it has four of them! (Figure 3.12).

This has important consequences for our goal of trying to recover wavelength information based on the responses of our photopigments. Yes, each photopigment's response depends on wavelength and intensity, so trying to just use one kind of photoreceptor won't allow us to make guesses about wavelength. However, by considering how different kinds of photoreceptors (specifically different kinds of cones) responded to the same light, we start to accumulate enough information to make better guesses about the ingredients of incoming light in terms of wavelength. To be more concrete about this, imagine that you knew your medium-wavelength cone had produced an intermediate response to some light: Not too large, but also not too small. What wavelength or wavelengths of light gave rise to that? Considered alone, it's very difficult to say: It could have been some dim light at this cell's peak sensitivity, or it could have been a much more intense light somewhere away from this peak. Without more information, we simply can't say. What if I told you that I also knew that the long-wavelength cones had a large response to this light and the short-wavelength cones had a small response, though? Now you can start to rule out some possibilities! In particular, it might be starting to sound like this light was rich in longer wavelengths and poor in shorter ones, which is more than we knew at first. We won't delve into the mathematics of how specific we can be about our guesses based on the three photoreceptor responses, but there are two big ideas I want to leave you with before we depart from the retina for destinations further along: (1) The different kinds of photoreceptor in your retina make it possible for you to infer wavelength content even though intensity is a confounding factor; (2) Those inferences are NOT perfect!

If you think back to your observations in the Spectroscopy exercise, you already saw evidence for my second point. If you recall, I asked you to take a look at some different kinds of light that all looked white to you and compare the emission spectra that you observed from each one. What you should have been able to see is that different light spectra (with different wavelengths) can still look white to you. Colors like this are referred to as metamers – physically different light sources that are perceptually indistinguishable – and they are a direct consequence of the limitations on our ability to use the photoreceptors to constrain our guesses about wavelength content. The number, location, and shape of our photoreceptors' absorption spectra determine the scope of what we can do to assign different subjective experiences to different combinations of light wavelengths and intensities. The colors that you can tell apart from one another depend on the inevitable numerical confusions that result from using photopigment responses this way to try and work backwards from retinal signals to light out in the world.

There are many, many interesting things to say about wavelength encoding at the retina that are beyond the scope of our observational approach to human vision, but I at least want to hint at some of them before we move on. In particular, I feel like I'd be remiss if I didn't point out that the ideas I described above offer important insights into the nature of color-blindness, a form of individual differences in wavelength encoding that is common in the general population. Behaviorally, color-blindness refers to a simple functional limitation: Individuals with color-blindness can't tell as many colors apart as other people. The source of this limitation is now easy for us to understand: Individuals with color-blindness either (1) Lack one or more of the three types of cones, or (2) Have cone absorption spectra that are shifted or shaped differently than other people. In the first case, which we refer to as either *monochromatism* or *dichromatism* depending on how many cones are unavailable, the limitation on color perception is due to having less information available to infer wavelength from photoreceptor responses. Three cones offer more constraints on our guesses than two, so missing a type of cone means that there are more possibilities for the kind of light that gave rise to your cells' responses. This means more *metamers* and more lights that look the same despite being physically different. In the second case, which we refer to as *anomalous* color vision, the difficulty arises from having too much redundant information – the shifted absorption spectrum of some of the cones means that the responses of different cones are more similar to one another, which means you get less independent information about incoming light. Again, this leads to more possibilities for what kind of light led to the cells' responses and, you guessed it, more metamers. In both cases, the increase in metamers means that there are more colors that look alike to the observer which increases color

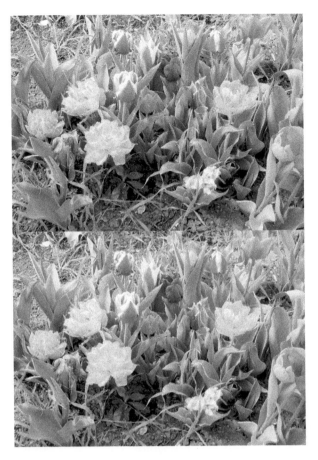

Figure 3.13 An individual with all three cone types would be able to see a wide variety of colors in this scene based on the different responses across the short, medium, and long wavelength cones. By comparison, not having the long wavelength cones available means that differences between incoming lights in terms of wavelength content are limited to what you can do by evaluating the two cones that are left. This limits the potential for different responses across some lights, leading to more colors that look the same. Image credit: Albarubescens, CC BY-SA 4.0 <https://creativecommons.org/licenses/by-sa/4.0/> via Wikimedia Commons.

confusion. In Figure 3.13, you can see what this means for someone who lacks their long-wavelength cone.

Our model retina clued us into some important aspects of how our visual system turns incoming light into a neural signal. It also helped us see how our experience is limited by the data we have available from our cells, which is in turn limited by their response properties. As we move along, this theme will only be more important to pay attention to – visual experience depends on working backwards from signals to estimates of the environment, so paying close attention to what we measure and how we can use it will be extremely important.

References

Anstis, S. (2010). Visual filling-in. *Current Biology: CB, 20*(16), R664–R666. https://doi.org/10.1016/j.cub.2010.06.029

Bradley, A., Zhang, H., Applegate, R. A., Thibos, L. N., & Elsner, A. E. (1998). Entoptic image quality of the retinal vasculature. *Vision Research, 38*(17), 2685–2696. https://doi.org/10.1016/s0042-6989(97)00345-3

Thibos, L., Lenner, K., & Thibos, C. (2023). Carl Bergmann (1814-1865) and the discovery of the anatomical site in the retina where vision is initiated. *Journal of the History of the Neurosciences,* 1–24. Advance online publication. https://doi.org/10.1080/0964704X.2023.2286991

4 Spatial Vision in the LGN and V1

Following wavelength encoding by the retina, information is sent onward to the next stages of visual processing along a pathway called the *geniculostriate pathway*. This pathway includes multiple anatomical structures including the layer of retinal ganglion cells in the eye, the layered structure of the lateral geniculate nucleus (LGN) in the thalamus, and the primary visual cortex (V1) in the occipital lobe. All three of those stages involve measuring some new properties of the patterns of light that have been projected across the surface of the retina: these are the subject of this chapter.

Specifically, the next steps in seeing involve the measurement of local contrast (the difference between nearby light and dark parts of an image) by the retinal ganglion cells, the lateral geniculate, and primary visual cortex. Each of these stages of visual processing is characterized in terms of the receptive field properties of the cells found in each place. Compared to the photoreceptors, we will be exploring how cells in these regions have excitatory and inhibitory regions within their receptive fields that govern how each type of cell will respond to different patterns of light and dark regions in the visual field. In the **Seeing Center-Surround Responses** lab, you will use a pattern called the Hermann grid (Spillman, 1994) to see some of the consequences of measuring local contrast the way cells in the LGN do and even measure some of those cell's properties psychophysically. We further explore how cells in different parts of the LGN contribute to visual experience by testing the different limits of **Central vs. Peripheral Vision** with regard to spatial acuity and color sensitivity. Next, we examine the nature of orientation selectivity in the primary visual cortex via the **Orientation Filtering** lab and follow this up with a measurement of **Instant Contrast Sensitivity**. Together, these exercises should give you insights into what each of these stages of visual processing measures about patterns of light and how that contributes to your visual experience of different images (Figure 4.1).

Testing Central vs. Peripheral Vision – How the Connections between the Photoreceptors and the Next Steps in Seeing Limit What You Can See Where

As we move beyond the layer of photoreceptors that we explored in our previous chapter, the measurements made by the rods and cones are sent onward to another class of cells that we call *retinal ganglion cells*. These cells are still inside the retina but receive signals from the photoreceptors that first transduce incoming light. On the basis of the anatomical connections between the photoreceptors and the ganglion cells alone, there are a few important observations we can make that have consequences for what we can see in different parts of our visual field.

DOI: 10.4324/9781032691169-5

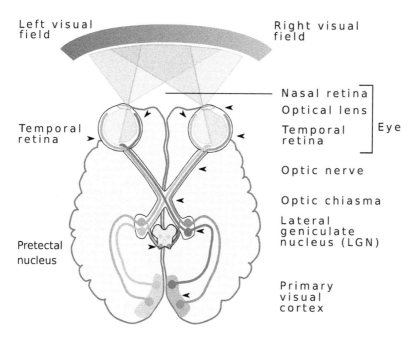

Figure 4.1 From the retina, signals are sent onward to the occipital lobe along the pathway displayed in this diagram. Information from the left and right visual field is ultimately processed by loci in the opposite hemispheres of the brain at the level of the lateral geniculate nucleus (LGN) and primary visual cortex (V1). Image credit: Miquel Perello Nieto, CC BY-SA 4.0 <https://creativecommons.org/licenses/by-sa/4.0>, via Wikimedia Commons.

In particular, compared to the rods and cones, there are far fewer retinal ganglion cells overall: The human eye has around 100 million photoreceptors, but there are only about one million retinal ganglion cells. This means that as information is being sent from the photoreceptors to the ganglion cells, there is a great deal of *convergence*. Information from multiple photoreceptors ends up being sent to the same ganglion cell. On average, the numbers I just mentioned imply about a 10:1 convergence ratio, but this turns out to vary by a lot depending on where we are in the retina. If we're looking at the fovea (the center of the retina), this convergence ratio might be more like 3:1 or 5:1, which means that just a few photoreceptors send information to the same ganglion cell. On the other hand, if we're looking at a part of the retina that's very far away from the fovea we could be looking at ratios more like hundreds or thousands to one! You can see a schematic diagram of what different amounts of convergence looks like in Figure 4.2. Remember from our previous chapter that the rods and cones are distributed very differently from one another across the fovea and the periphery, with cones being densely packed into the fovea and rods dominating in the periphery.

This big difference in the anatomy between the center of the retina and its periphery has an equally big impact on what you can see in the center of your visual field compared to the edges. In this next set of exercises, we'll test your vision in a few simple ways to compare what you can see when you're looking right at different stimuli to what you can see when those same images are even just a little bit out to the sides of your visual field (Figure 4.3).

Low Convergence   **High Convergence**

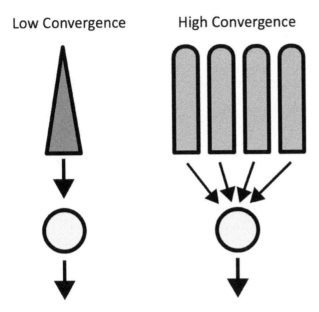

Figure 4.2 Between the retina and the LGN there are varying amounts of convergence such that information from many cells is all sent to the same destination in some parts of the visual field, while elsewhere only a few cells send information to the same downstream neuron. This varying convergence has substantial consequences for our visual function in central vs. peripheral vision. Image credit: Photo by the author.

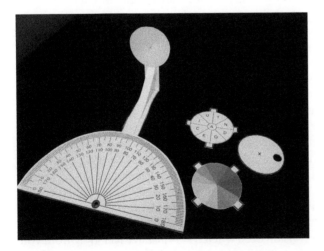

Figure 4.3 We can test visual acuity at different parts of the visual field with a simple testing procedure and a supporting apparatus (if necessary). Photo by the author.

Things you will need:

- A Landolt C printed on a piece of paper or cardstock.
- A collection of LEGO bricks, crayons, or other easily carried colorful objects.
- A protractor, OR
- A printable peripheral vision testing apparatus (included in the supplementary material available with the textbook).

Testing Central Visual Acuity

Start by cutting out the Landolt C pattern and testing a partner's visual acuity using this "staircase" method: Stand a few feet from them and rotate the C to one of the cardinal directions (N,S,E and W) or an intermediate angle (NW, NE, SW, SE). If they get the answer correct, take a step backwards, reorient the C at random, and try again. If they get the answer wrong, take a step forward and do the same – turn the C to a new direction at random and ask them which way it's pointing. If you keep doing this, you should be able to find a *threshold*, a place where moving just a little further tends to make the C too small to see, but moving just a little closer makes it easy. One simple way to decide when you've reached this threshold is to stop after they make a certain number of mistakes (maybe five or six). However you decide to determine this value, measure how far away you are from your partner when you reach it.

Testing Peripheral Visual Acuity

Repeat the exercise above, but with a different staircase: Sit a fixed distance from your partner with the C in front of them (I'd recommend about five feet or so) and adjust where the C is in the visual periphery depending on whether or not they get the orientation of the letter correct. You can use a protractor to help you be consistent if you like, but it's also ok if you're estimating how much closer or further you move the pattern towards the center of their visual field. They key is to move a little closer to their central vision if they get the answer wrong and move a little further away if they get the answer right. Just like in the previous exercise, you should be able to identify a threshold distance where you bounce back and forth between your partner making mistakes and your partner getting the answer correct. How far away from the center of their visual field is this threshold distance if you sit five feet away from your partner? What about if you sit ten feet away from them?

What I hope you were able to see (or perhaps not see!) in these tests is that there is a big difference between your acuity in the central part of your visual field and even just a little distance away from it. My guess is that when you and your partner were allowed to look right at the letter C, that threshold distance where you just started to make mistakes was pretty far away – I've had students end up all the way at the end of long hallways when they do this experiment in my classes! On the other hand, I bet that the letter C was quite difficult to see clearly out your peripheral vision even when it was just five feet away from you.

This difference in acuity is directly related to those big differences in convergence between the photoreceptors and ganglion cells in the central and peripheral parts of your retina. To think about why this is the case, I want you to imagine that you're going to try and figure out where light came from in the visual field by paying attention to a single retinal ganglion cell: If it produces a signal, you'll know light must have landed on the photoreceptors that it's connected to. If it doesn't, you'll know there wasn't enough light on those photoreceptors to make this ganglion cell produce its own signal. If the ganglion cell we're listening to is connected to just 3–5 photoreceptors, once we see it begin signaling we can make a pretty good guess about where light must have been on the retina. Light had to be somewhere in that little group of photoreceptors that are connected to our cell! On the other hand, if the ganglion cell we're listening to is connected to hundreds or thousands of photoreceptors, our job is a lot harder: Activity in our ganglion cell could mean light was in lots of different places over the part of the retina where those thousands of photoreceptors are arranged. We'll be able to guess that the light landed on the retina somewhere in that neighborhood, but it's a big, big neighborhood!

The difference between being able to make a precise guess (or *inference*) about where light must have been on the retina and being stuck with a vague guess is what you're experiencing when you try to measure where the gap is in the Landolt C in different parts of your visual field. The inability to be precise about where light came from after we send signals to the retinal ganglion cells leads patterns of light and dark in the periphery to look less distinct. However, an advantage of that high convergence that we didn't test in this experiment is that it tends to make you more sensitive to detecting small amounts of light in your peripheral vision compared to central vision. Having thousands of photoreceptors all sending signals to a single ganglion cell isn't so good for being precise about exactly where light was, but it also means you have thousands of chances to at least send along the information that there was some light.

In our next set of visual tests, we're going to look at one more difference between central and peripheral vision that depends on the convergence of photoreceptors onto retinal ganglion cells: Your color sensitivity across the visual field.

Testing Chromatic Sensitivity

In this exercise, you're going to measure another kind of threshold in central vision compared to peripheral vision. We're not going to use a spatial pattern of light the way we did with the Landolt C however, because we're not examining how sensitive you are to differences in where light and dark parts of an image are this time. Instead, we're going to ask how sensitive you are to differences in color at different parts of your visual field.

To do this, you'll use the colored pencils, crayons, or LEGO bricks to do a color-naming exercise. It doesn't matter a great deal what kind of colored objects you use, but I'd suggest getting something that's small enough to hold in your hand and that comes in enough colors for you to have at least five or six possibilities to show your partner. In a pinch, you can cut out small squares of construction paper, or make something like the color wheel included in the supplementary material. Whichever objects you choose, repeat the staircase tasks that we did before by showing your partner a random color that they get to look directly at and asking them to name it. Just like before, take a step further away if they're right and take a step closer if they're wrong. My guess is that you're going to get very, very far away from them again before they make five or six mistakes! Once you've done that, repeat the staircase exercise we did with peripheral vision using these objects, too: Sit about five feet away from your partner, and start by showing them a random object in their central vision and asking them to name it. If they get the answer right, move a little bit away from their central vision and, if they get it wrong, move a little bit closer. My guess is that you won't have to get far before they start having some serious problems guessing what color you're holding up.

The difference in color sensitivity that you should have been able to see here also depends on those connections between the photoreceptors and the retinal ganglion cells. Besides the overall differences in convergence that we see in the central part of the retina compared to the periphery, there are also differences in exactly which photoreceptors are sending signals to which ganglion cells depending on where we are in the retina. Specifically, those retinal ganglion cells in the central part of the retina tend to have their connections from photoreceptors arranged in a very particular way: They tend to have connections from just one kind of cone (let's say a "red" cone that is most sensitive to long wavelengths of light) positioned in one part of the retina and connections from another kind of cone (maybe a "green" cone that is most sensitive to medium wavelengths of light) from a part of the retina *around* the first region. This organization is called a *center-surround* structure and it makes it possible for the activity of this ganglion cell to tell us something specific about not just where the light came from one the retina, but what *kind* of light (by which we mean wavelengths and color) it was. You can see what that center-surround architecture looks like in Figure 4.4.

For the moment, don't worry so much about what it means to have these connections separated spatially by red vs. green cones. We'll get to that in our next exercise. For now, the important idea is that the retinal ganglion cells in the central part of your retina keep information from different kinds of cones separate, which makes it possible to measure differences in the wavelengths of light falling on different parts of the retina that they are connected to. By comparison, the retinal ganglion cells in the peripheral part of the retina not only have much larger convergence (many more photoreceptors connecting to them) but they also don't keep the information from different kinds of cones organized or separated in the same way as the cells in central vision. Because these cells only get information from all three types of cones throughout the part of the retina they're connected to, or only get information from rod photoreceptors, there isn't a way to measure differences in the wavelengths of light that are landing on different parts of the retina.

These aren't the only ways in which your peripheral vision differs from your central vision (see Strasburger et al., 2011, for an extensive review), but hopefully this gives you some intuition regarding the way in which anatomical features of your visual system end up having direct functional consequences that constrain what you can and can't see under different circumstances. We'll continue by examining what the pattern of connections across retinal space means for the patterns you see in the visual field in our next exercise, which will move us onward from the retinal ganglion cell layer to a structure called the *lateral geniculate nucleus*.

Seeing Center-Surround Responses with the Hermann Grid

To continue examining how the structure of receptive fields in our next stages of vision determines what we measure and experience about patterns of light, we will look more closely at this idea of center-surround structure in cells that are part of the retinal ganglion layer and the lateral geniculate nucleus. Remember that the former is a layer of cells in the retina that pool information from the photoreceptors before sending signals along the optic nerve to the visual brain, while the latter is a structure in the *thalamus* that receives those connections.

The distinctions that we have already made between central and peripheral vision continue at these stages of visual processing, and are in some ways defined even more clearly by the anatomy of both regions. The lateral geniculate nucleus in particular is a layered

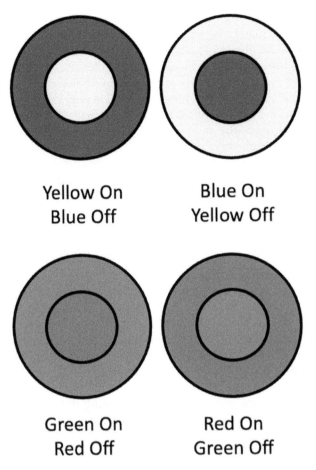

Yellow On
Blue Off

Blue On
Yellow Off

Green On
Red Off

Red On
Green Off

Figure 4.4 Some cells receive inputs from the photoreceptors such that responses from different types of photoreceptors change the way the cell responds to light that was in different parts of the visual field. For example, some cells may have excitatory connections between long-wavelength cones and the central part of their receptive field along with inhibitory connections between medium-wavelength cones and the outer ring of their receptive field. This means that these cells are capable of responding based on color contrast, contributing to your ability to distinguish colors. Illustration by the author.

structure (six layers in total) that is organized in a manner that segregates some of the different modes of visual processing we introduced in the retina. If we consider the retinal ganglion cells which had very high convergence, for example, with a very large number of photoreceptors sending connections to a single retinal ganglion cell, these make connections to the lower two layers of the LGN. We call these the *magnocellular layers* to reflect the large size of the receptive field associated with these cells and also the large size of the dendritic arbor of each cell that we find here. Turning our attention to those cells in the retinal ganglion layer that had low convergence (just a few photoreceptors connecting to each cell), these make connections in the upper four layers of the LGN, which we call the *parvocellular layers*. Remember that we said these low-convergence retinal ganglion cells

tended to organize connections from different kinds of cones spatially within their receptive fields, making it possible to measure information about the different wavelengths of
light that landed on different parts of the retina. Cells in the parvocellular layer of the LGN
inherit this capability, while the cells in the magnocellular layer are not able to provide
much information about wavelength. Instead, these cells only signal differences in light
intensity (bright vs. dark appearance) across different parts of their receptive fields.

What these cells across all six layers of the LGN share, however, is a functional architecture that makes it possible to start measuring patterns of light in the visual field. Regardless
of whether we are talking about the magnocellular or parvocellular layer, the cells in the
lateral geniculate nucleus measure contrast between a central circular region in the receptive field and an annulus surrounding that central dot. This is achieved by combining an
excitatory portion of the cell's receptive field (a region in which more light will increase
the likelihood that the cell produces a signal) with an inhibitory portion (a region in which
more light will instead decrease the likelihood that a cell produces a signal). An arrangement of excitatory and inhibitory regions in a receptive field that includes a central dot
with an annulus (or ring) around it is referred to as *Center-Surround* structure. Critically,
such a receptive field will not produce a signal if the receptive field is filled with uniform
light. Such a stimulus would pit the excitatory region directly against the inhibitory region,
leading to nothing at all. Instead, these cells produce signals in response to patterns that
include local increments or decrements in luminance or color. This is the first step in
encoding something about the spatial arrangement of different light intensities and wavelengths across the visual field. Moreover, the activity of these cells is the basis for what you
see – this is what we will explore here. The structure of these receptive fields makes some
patterns capable of driving strong responses in these cells and other patterns less capable
of doing so, leading to some surprising outcomes in patterns like the Hermann grid. In
this exercise, you will use variations on the grid pattern as a tool for testing the explana-
tory power of center-surround cells as an account of our perception of these simple images
(Figure 4.5).

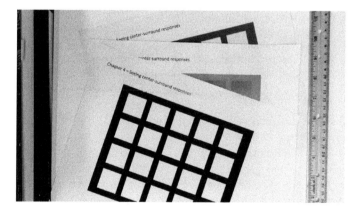

Figure 4.5 Grid-like patterns allow us to see evidence of the selectivity of lateral geniculate nucleus
cells for bright and dark spots as well as color contrast relationships. With some simple
measurements, we can even start to characterize the size of receptive fields in different
parts of the visual field. Photo by the author.

Things you will need:

- The grayscale and color Hermann grids included in the supplementary material (or you can easily make your own).
- A tape measure or ruler.

Observing Illusory Dots in Central and Peripheral Vision

Start by looking at the grayscale grid with dark squares and bright roads. We are going to use this pattern to tell a bit of a story about how cells with center-surround structure should respond to different parts of this image and use that to try and explain some things that we see when we look at it. Remember that when we talk about excitatory and inhibitory parts of a receptive field, we are talking about parts of the receptive field where more light makes a cell more likely to respond (excitatory region) and other parts of the receptive field where more light will make a cell less likely to respond (inhibitory region). The arrangement of these regions within a cell determines what kind of light pattern within the receptive field will produce the largest response from the cell.

The neat thing about the patterns we will use here is the following (and this applies to all of the different versions of the grid provided here): The response of a center-surround cell positioned with its central region at the junction of two roads is different than that same cell's response if its central region instead lands within a single road. This is because of how much of the surrounding annulus ends up taken up by light. In the case of what we call an ON-Center cell (a cell with a central excitatory region, see Figure 4.6), a cell at the crossroads is inhibited more by the multiple bright roads landing in the surround than a cell centered within a single road and only two intrusions of light into the outer ring (Figure 4.6).

The result is that the response of that cell at the crossroads will tend to be lower than the response of the cell within a single road. These cells' activity is an indicator of local luminance increments. That is, an ON-center cell's response is a key factor in signaling to your visual system that there is a bright spot at some part of the visual field. A differential response between different ON-center cells should mean that you have a different experience of how bright things look in the portions of the visual field being measured by those cells. In this case, our diagram in Figure 4.6 implies that the junctions should look a little darker than the middle of the roads, which you should experience as fuzzy gray dots at those junctions! Confirm that you can see these with the two grayscale patterns, reflecting both ON-Center and OFF-Center activity (at least according to our account of what's happening here). Remember: Those fuzzy dots are not there in a physical sense, but are meaningful in terms of the signals being sent by the cells at this stage of visual processing.

Quantifying Illusory Dot Appearance in Central and Peripheral Vision

The cells in the LGN vary in size depending on their position in either the parvocellular or magnocellular layers of this structure and depending on where they are within each of those layers. Cells that receive input from central vision tend to have smaller receptive fields, while cells receiving input from peripheral vision are larger. Because these illusory dots depend on the center-surround structure of the cells' receptive fields, this means there is a size-dependency to this effect. Confirm this by looking at a particular fuzzy dot, then moving it closer to your face until the dot disappears. What is the critical distance for the

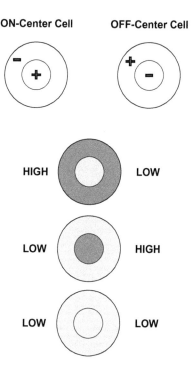

Figure 4.6 Schematic diagrams of how cells in the retinal ganglion layer and LGN with center-surround structure would respond to various patterns of light. ON-center cells will produce a strong response to a small spot of light in the very center of the receptive field, while OFF-center cells will respond strongly when there is much more light in the surrounding annulus. Neither cell responds especially much when light fills the entire receptive field as the inhibitory and excitatory signals largely cancel one another out. Illustration by the author.

dots to be visible in the grayscale patterns? Repeat this exercise with a dot in the periphery. Which peripheral dots are visible at a given viewing distance? What is the eccentricity (the distance out to the sides of your visual field) of those dots? Use your tape measure and your protractor to help answer these questions.

Chromatic Center-Surround Responses

Finally repeat these exercises with each of the chromatic Hermann grids to see how color contrast may operate differently than grayscale contrast. In the LGN, cells responsive to chroma vs. luminance occupy different layers of the LGN and also have some differences in receptive field size. Does this lead to different critical distances and eccentricities for seeing the illusory dots?

The "Classical" Account of the Hermann Grid vs. Some Easy-To-Observe Problems with It.

So far, I hope I've presented you with a decent argument that we can understand why we do and don't see these illusory fuzzy dots in the Hermann grid so long as we understand how these center-surround cells respond to different configurations of light. This is a nice look at how we can link some properties of what individual cells are doing at different stages of visual processing directly to our visual experience. The key idea here is that what you see depends in a surprisingly direct way on the properties of the cells at different stages of the visual system. Perhaps more importantly, what you experience of the visual world is not a perfect reflection of what is actually in the environment. In this case, you experienced a simple illusion that we can explain using the properties of cells in the LGN that measure spatial patterns of light. To put it another way, we were able to think through how your visual experience was really a reflection of the activity produced in these cells by the environment rather than an accurate record of the environment itself. This means that understanding what patterns of light are being measured by different cells in early stages of vision is an important step towards explaining why we see many of the things that we do.

This would be a wonderful place to stop if not for one small problem: The story I have presented to you is known to be wrong!

Well, "wrong" is perhaps too strong a word. Let's say instead that it is too limited. If this is the case, why did I bother telling you all this stuff then? The answer is that I think the successes and the failures of this classical account of the Hermann grid offer an especially valuable opportunity to see how we can use simple observations to both develop, test, and refine these kinds of explanations for different visual phenomena. In closing this experiment, I want to give you a chance to see just one of the key limits of this classical story about these fuzzy dots.

Here is a simple test of our theory as presented so far: Those center-surround cells are circular, so they shouldn't change what they're doing if we spin the Hermann grid around, right? As far as the center-surround cells are concerned, they get the same distribution of light and dark stuff inside their receptive field however we rotate this pattern, so the fuzzy dots should stay the same as we spin the Hermann grid. The trouble is that, if you turn the grid so that the roads are diagonal (let's say 45 degrees or so), you will likely see that the fuzzy dots are less distinct! If we introduce some other small changes to the pattern that also keep the light/dark material in the receptive fields of these cells the same (for example, using wavy roads instead of straight ones), we find that those changes also greatly diminish the illusory effect (Geier et al., 2008).

On one hand, maybe this feels like a disappointment. Do we actually know how this illusion works at all? I want to argue that this is actually really exciting. We were able to use a fairly simple set of facts to account for something that we saw, and then we were able to make more observations *with the same piece of paper* that helped us see that we needed something else to explain those new observations. Reader: *That* is vision science in perhaps its purest form. As we continue, a lot of what I will have to offer you in subsequent chapters are indeed partial or incomplete accounts of the data. The exciting thing about vision science, though, is how readily available new data is and how many anatomical and functional facts we have to build upon as we try to explain more and more about why things look the way that they do to us. We'll continue by introducing a few more properties of the cells in early stages of visual processing and thinking about how the properties of those cells also determine what we can see.

Orientation Filtering with Lenticular Film

Our next step in visual processing after the LGN is the primary visual cortex, also known as area V1. While the cells in the LGN respond to patterns of light with a center-surround structure, the cells in V1 are sensitive to a different kind of pattern: Oriented lines and edges. This is achieved by arranging the excitatory and inhibitory regions of these cell's receptive fields in different configurations than the center-surround structure we described before. A typical V1 cell might have a central vertical strip that is excitatory, flanked by inhibitory vertical strips to the left and right. A cell with this kind of receptive field would produce strong responses to bright vertical lines on a dark background. Different cells in V1 are tuned to different orientations of light/dark edges via different arrangements of these excitatory and inhibitory regions within their receptive field. This means that within the primary visual cortex there are sub-populations of cells that primarily respond to the horizontal edges in a scene, while other cells will primarily respond to the vertical edges in a scene, and so on for many different orientations of lines and edges.

One way to think about what is happening at this stage of visual processing is to consider each of these sub-populations as a different channel of visual information that will include some structures in the visual environment and omit others. To see what this is like, we'll use lenticular film in this exercise to see how orientation filters make some features in a visual scene more prominent depending on how oriented edges are distributed in the environment.

Things you will need:

- A sheet of lenticular film. This can be a little difficult to find, but all you really need is a piece that is about 20cm × 20cm.
- Colored pencils or crayons.
- Some interesting pictures of objects/scenes.

Horizontal and Vertical Orientation Filtering in a Schematic Scene

We'll start by looking at how lenticular film can be selective for orientation in much the same way as a sub-population of V1 cells might be. Begin by arranging a bunch of crayons in a loose pile (see Figure 4.7) with different crayons tilted in different directions. Ideally you should have crayons pointing lots of different ways.

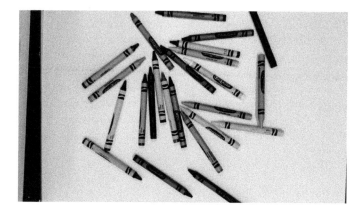

Figure 4.7 Begin by scattering some crayons on a surface so that they are tilted in many different directions. Photo by the author.

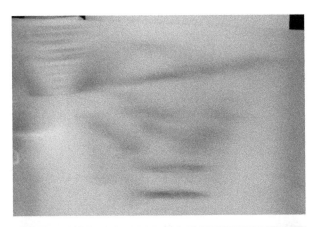

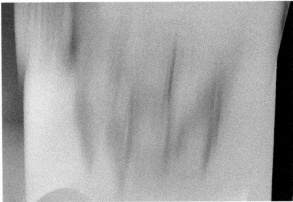

Figure 4.8 By varying the orientation of the lenticular film, you can see what aspects of the image are visible when only some orientation information is allowed to pass through the film. Photo by the author.

Lenticular film has long grooves in it that make light diffuse differently along and across those grooves. Look at your pile of crayons with those grooves oriented vertically, then turn the film so that they are oriented horizontally. This should lead you to see only the crayons that are oriented in one direction or the other (Figure 4.8).

Horizontal and Vertical Orientation Filtering in a Naturalistic Scene

Now let's see what this is like in a more complex natural image. I've just selected a photo from a magazine in Figure 4.9, but you can use whatever you like. Regardless of your choice, hold the lenticular film just above the image with the columns oriented horizontally and vertically and note the difference in appearance (Figure 4.9).

If possible, it's worth trying this with specific types of objects or images to see how different kinds of information occupy different orientation channels. Faces, for example, tend to be much more recognizable when the horizontal information is present than when the vertical information is all you can see (Dakin & Watt, 2009). Bodies tend to be just

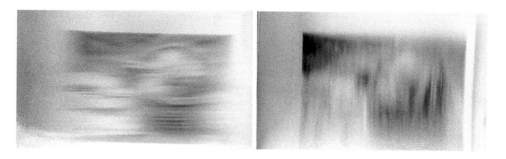

Figure 4.9 Repeating this exercise with a complex image allows us to assess what orientations contribute the most to different recognition judgments. Photo by the author.

the opposite, however (Balas et al., 2018), so a horizontal filter can make pedestrians in a street scene nearly vanish. Even though we're still talking about early stages of visual processing, the nature of these measurements has consequences for everything that comes later. Recognizing people, determining how to pick something up based on its shape, and any other complex visual task is based on this suite of measurements of unoriented contrast (in the LGN) and oriented contrast (in V1).

Instant Contrast Sensitivity Testing

Before we leave these early stages of visual processing for destinations that are further along and that offer more complex kinds of computation about our visual environment, it's worth examining what kind of spatial vision the cells in the LGN and V1 provide us with. We've seen that cells in the LGN are sensitive to the size of spatial patterns with the right structure for their receptive fields, while the cells in V1 are sensitive to both size and orientation. I need to introduce an important term of art right now and tell you that when we're talking about size and contrast in the manner that LGN and V1 cells measure it, vision scientists tend to use the term *spatial frequency*. This term is used because it is often useful to think about size and scale in images in terms of the alternation between light and dark within some amount of space: If there are many alternations between light and dark within some part of an image, we could say this is an example of a high spatial frequency pattern. On the other hand, if there are very few alternations between light and dark within the same part of an image, we would call this an example of a low spatial frequency pattern.

Your ability to see visual structures at greater or lesser levels of detail depends in part on the population of LGN and V1 cells that you have and their ability to send signals about patterns with varying spatial frequency. One way we can quantify your spatial vision with regard to spatial frequency is to measure something called the *contrast sensitivity function* (CSF). This is a curve that describes the amount of contrast you need between the lightest and darkest parts of an image to distinguish stripes with a particular spatial frequency from a uniform gray image. This is different than measuring your visual acuity and can provide valuable information for diagnosing various kinds of diseases that affect vision (Richman et al., 2013). Measuring this full curve is typically a time-consuming and tedious procedure but provides a rich description of the capabilities of your visual system in terms of seeing different kinds of spatial patterns. We would like to get a glimpse of this rich description in this exercise, but you probably don't have the time for a full measurement of the CSF. To get around this practical limitation, we are going to *cheat*.

Things you will need:

- An 8.5" × 11" printout of stripes with spatial frequency varying on the x-axis and contrast varying on the y-axis. (See the supplementary material for a version of this pattern you can print out.)
- Some transparencies.
- A dry-erase marker.

Measuring Individual Contrast Sensitivity Instantly

What we're interested in is how well you can see a light/dark alternation as (1) spatial frequency changes and (2) contrast increases or decreases. The image in Figure 4.10 will be our tool for doing so as it depicts light/dark stripes that grow increasingly closer together as we move left-to-right (decreasing spatial frequency) and that grow increasingly faint as we move bottom-to-top (decreasing contrast). What we want to know is when you stop seeing the stripes at each spatial frequency. Place your transparency on top of this image, keep your head a fixed distance away from it, and use the dry-erase marker to draw the boundary between stripes and gray stuff from left-to-right across the image (Figure 4.11).

Most people will find that the line rises to a peak in the middle of the picture, then declines slowly as you continue to the right. This reflects your visual system's maximal sensitivity to intermediate spatial frequencies, with less of your V1 population sending signals

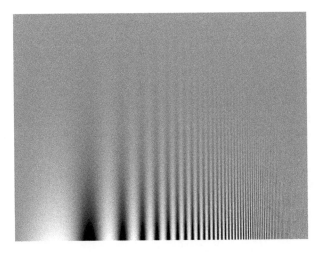

Figure 4.10 We can quickly measure your contrast sensitivity function using the pattern depicted here, dry-erase markers, and a bit of transparent film. Photo by the author.

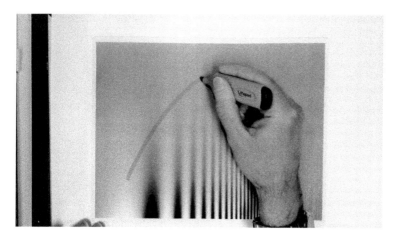

Figure 4.11 Quickly assess your own contrast threshold for different spatial frequencies by deciding
the height at which the black-and-white stripes fade to gray. Photo by the author.

about either very coarse or very fine edges. Your mileage may vary, however, which is why
it's a good idea to ask more than one person.

Aggregating CSF Measurements across Observers

Repeat the procedure above with a bunch of people, ideally each with their own transparency and dry-erase marker. If you decide to try this out, it's worth adding a mark for the
corner of the CSF image to the transparency so you know how to line up all the responses
after everyone is done. Doing this with enough people should allow you to overlay the
different CSF curves for your observers to see what the group thinks they can see. Here's
a version done via Zoom with my class (Figure 4.12).

This is a handy way to quickly get a sense of the limits of your spatial vision without spending too much of your life in a psychophysical testing suite. For some added
insight, try rotating the pattern so that the lines are horizontal or diagonal and see if the
curve changes at all. Your primary visual cortex has more horizontal and vertical cells than
oblique ones, which may be reflected in your sensitivity to those orientations. In any event,
this curve is a nice summary of the range your early visual system provides you with for
measuring different kinds of light/dark patterns in natural images. If you're remembering
what we said about the different layers of the LGN, you might be wondering what happened to processing color, but that's still happening too! You have CSFs for different color
contrasts as well as for light/dark contrast, all of which are a function of the properties
of the cells you have in these stages of visual processing. Again, the key idea to take away
from this chapter is that you don't see what is out in the world, you see the responses of
the cells that you use to measure what is out in the world. In the next chapters, we'll run
into this idea again and again, each time with regard to a different kind of visual problem
that we'd like to solve.

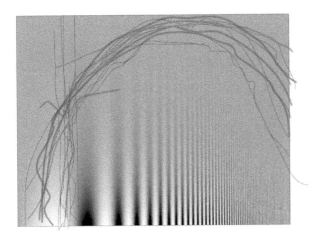

Figure 4.12 Estimates from several students in my class that reveal the typical shape of the contrast sensitivity function. Try varying the orientation of the pattern to see how it might change. Photo by the author.

References

Balas, B., Auen, A., Saville, A., & Schmidt, J. (2018). Body emotion recognition disproportionately depends on vertical orientations during childhood. *International Journal of Behavioral Development, 42*(2), 278–283. https://doi.org/10.1177/0165025417690267

Dakin, S. C., & Watt, R. J. (2009). Biological "bar codes" in human faces. *Journal of Vision, 9*(4), 1–10. https://doi.org/10.1167/9.4.2

Geier, J., Bernáth, L., Hudák, M., & Séra, L. (2008). Straightness as the main factor of the Hermann grid illusion. *Perception, 37,* 651–665.

Richman, J., Spaeth, G. L., & Wirostko, B. (2013). Contrast sensitivity basics and a critique of currently available tests. *Journal of Cataract and Refractive Surgery, 39*(7), 1100–1106. https://doi.org/10.1016/j.jcrs.2013.05.001

Spillmann, L. (1994). The hermann grid illusion: A tool for studying human perceptive field organization. *Perception, 23,* 691–708.

Strasburger, H., Rentschler, I., & Jüttner, M. (2011). Peripheral vision and pattern recognition: A review. *Journal of Vision, 11*(5), 13. https://doi.org/10.1167/11.5.13

5 Perceptual Organization and Gestalt Principles

Early stages of visual processing like those described in the previous chapter involve highly local measurements of contrast and independent channels for measuring chroma, luminance, spatial frequency, and orientation. To put it more simply, we've seen that the cells in the retinal ganglion layer, the LGN, and primary visual cortex make lots of measurements of patterns of light, leaving us with a description of incoming images in terms of lots of small pieces. If we think about the receptive field structures we experimented with in the last chapter, we have cells that measure spots of brightness and darkness, spots of color, and lines and edges tilted different directions, all of which are measured at different sizes. That's a lot of information, so what do we do with all of it to end up with our visual experience and our visual abilities?

This fragmented encoding of visual information eventually has to yield something more compact and capable of supporting the recognition of objects, the perception of surfaces and scenes, and a visual understanding of what we are looking at. *Perceptual organization* refers to the principles that govern the assemblage of pieces of visual structure into more meaningful wholes. How do we combine small elements of the visual world into more complicated ones? How do we determine when visual features should be split apart rather than grouped together? The Gestalt psychologists identified a number of these principles, most of which share a common theme of what they referred to as "pragnanz" or "good form." By this, we mean that the manner in which your visual system appears to group small elements of visual structure into larger forms favors grouping solutions that promote simplicity, regularity, and consistency with the occurrence of forms in the visual environment. If that seems like a somewhat hazy definition of what it means to have good form, then I'm afraid I'd have to agree with you. Though there has been progress in making the idea of pragnanz more explicit and quantitative, it is still challenging to summarize all of the grouping principles that your visual system uses into one comprehensive model. Our goal in this section is thus to build intuitions for what kinds of rules your visual system appears to use to group and segment smaller-scale visual features through some simple demonstrations of perceptual organization. By seeing what forms are apparent to you in different settings where perceptual organization is necessary, you should be able to start enumerating your own list of heuristics that human vision uses at this stage of processing.

In **Pragnanz Telephone** and **Metzger's Tiny Drawings**, we will use drawings made under impoverished conditions to examine what your visual system means by "good form" as an organizing principle that is used to account for incomplete data. Next, we will examine one particular aspect of good form in particular by investigating the nature of **Illusory volumes and surfaces** using simple inducing elements made from paper and designed to make it easy to test the limits of a process called amodal completion.

DOI: 10.4324/9781032691169-6

Pragnanz "Telephone"

You may already be familiar with the game of "Telephone" in which a large group of people passes a message from person to person via whispers in an effort to try to preserve the original message as accurately as possible. The fun part of this game, however, is comparing the message obtained at the end to the original message used at the beginning of the game. Misheard and misspoken words at any particular point in the communication chain can compound, leading to potentially large errors in transmitting the message and a final outcome that may differ in surprising ways from what you started with.

In this group exercise (first suggested to me by Dr. Cedar Riener), we'll use a game of visual telephone to crowdsource the heuristics used by a bunch of observers given noisy measurements of visual form. An important difference between the usual spoken game of Telephone and this version is that in this case we are not considering the errors made by each player to simply be a source of fun. Instead, we are critically interested in these mistakes! Our rationale is that whatever errors a particular player makes when attempting to reconstruct the patterns they saw are a reflection of how their visual system organized the input that they were presented with. While errors in spoken Telephone are interesting because they diverge from the original signal, in this game our assumption is that compounding errors across multiple participants may converge on properties of pragnanz shared by our players.

Things you will need:

- Some blank pieces of paper (one per student).
- Sharpies, pens, or other drawing implements.

Initializing the Gestalt Telephone

Begin by drawing a collection of scribbles on a piece of paper with your marker. These should be asymmetric, random, and messy. I've found it's especially good to include lines that don't quite meet up, lines that are not exactly parallel, and other sorts of imperfections that make the lines difficult to summarize with a succinct description. Place each discrete scribble randomly on the page as well – don't place your set of squiggles on the corners of an imaginary square, for example (Figure 5.1).

Placing Quick "Calls" with Your Set of Observers

This game is best played with a group of about 10–12 people, but fewer than this is probably enough to see some interesting things. Begin the game by showing your initial pattern to your first observer for just 2–3 seconds, then ask them to draw what they saw on their own sheet of paper. The limited amount of time obviously means that they will likely not have caught all of the details in your original drawing but ask them to do the best they can from their memory of what they saw. Once they've drawn what they can, they must show their drawing to the next observer for 2–3 seconds and this new person now draws the pattern as best as they can recall it. Continue as follows for all of your observers and then compare the initial drawing to the last one (see Figure 5.2).

You should find that the random, noisy squiggles you made at the beginning of the game rapidly gave way to forms that were different. In particular, you may find that the squiggles drawn by the last player included more symmetrical individual shapes, lines that were closer to parallel, lines that meet nicely at corners, and other aspects of pragnanz.

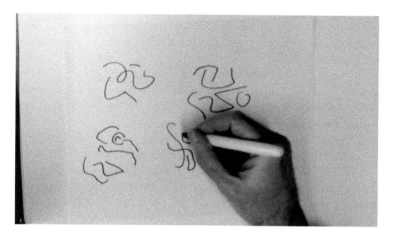

Figure 5.1 Draw a set of random shapes and lines at different positions on your paper to begin the exercise. Photo by the author.

How it started...   ...how it's going.

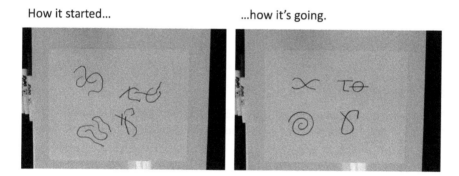

Figure 5.2 Compare your initial drawing to those made by students towards the end of the sequence. You are likely to see emergent symmetry, parallelism, tidier junctions, and other hallmarks of pragnanz. Photo by the author.

A few more specific elements to look at closely include the angles made by lines that meet up at some junction: Do these tend to be closer to angles like **60** or **90** degrees, for example? Likewise, if lines had variable spacing between them such that some were far apart and others were closer together, did this turn into more consistent spacing in the final drawing? Finally, if your original squiggles were positioned haphazardly on the page, where are the final squiggles positioned? In Figure 5.2, you can see that this group of players let the squiggles drift over the course of the game until they were indeed positioned at the corners of an approximate square. In some cases, you may even see that squiggles merge together after several players have had a chance to draw the patterns.

   Again, the key idea here is that the errors that emerge in the observers' drawings are actually reflections of the heuristics used to organize visual features into intermediate forms. To the extent that you see some of the same changes as those described above, this indicates your visual system's use of heuristics that favor symmetrical forms, uniformity in spacing, line weight, and other visual features, and the continuation of contours in a manner that promotes smoothness rather than abrupt changes in orientation. If you like, see how things change with more time given for each transmission of the image through the telephone line. This can help reveal what properties of the image are perceived with more fidelity quickly as compared to those that are reproduced with more emphasis on the underlying Gestalt principles of perceptual organization.

Metzger's "Tiny Drawings"

A game of visual Telephone is a fun way to examine principles of good form in a group setting but doesn't tell us much about what any one individual contributed. It also obviously requires a rather large group of people and takes a fair amount of time to complete. By comparison, this exercise is very similar to the last one, but is much faster and yields many of the same insights. Like our game of Telephone described in the previous section, we are still going to present observers with drawings that are difficult to see in all their complexity and use reproductions of these drawings as a way to identify the nature of pragnanz. Again, in this case the mistakes that we see are not just errors but are instead treated as the positive expression of the underlying heuristics used to organize our perception of complex scenes. The difference is that in this case we will not use viewing time as a means of reducing the fidelity of image perception but will instead use the size of a drawing as a different way to weaken observers' ability to see the idiosyncratic details of a complex shape. Rather than seeing the emergence of "good form" across a group of observers, this exercise requires each person to rely on their own internal sense of pragnanz to guide their recreation of the visual forms that they saw (Metzger, 2009).

Things you will need:

- Some blank pieces of paper (one per student).
- Sharpies, pens, or other drawing implements.

Much like the **Pragnanz Telephone** exercise, the idea here is to draw a set of irregular doodles that include misaligned contours, asymmetries, and other visual features that are not especially "nice" in terms of good form for students to draw under impoverished conditions. Begin by making a couple of drawings like this freehand or in your favorite graphics program (one of my few deviations from the analog theme of this book!) and then resize them to be really REALLY small. The idea is to give participants only a limited ability to really see what's in these doodles (Figure 5.3).

Figure 5.4 shows the original versions of some squiggles that I drew for this experiment in my own classroom. Note the various irregular contours, partially overlapping or not-quite-overlapping lines, and other such features that are not especially nice in terms of good form.

Here are those same drawings resized to be teensy. You may want to be a little careful with regard to line thickness and other properties of the resized drawings to give your participants enough visual structure to work with at all, but these are intended to be rather hard to see. Unlike the previous game of Pragnanz Telephone, participants should have as much time to see these tiny drawings as they would like – We are limiting the measurements you can carry out on these drawings with a spatial manipulation rather than a temporal one. Based on what you can see in this limited view, what do participants think

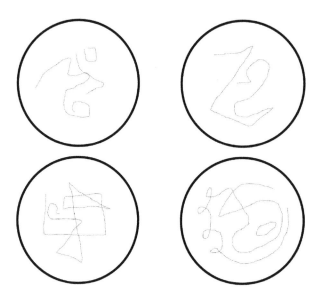

Figure 5.3 These are more random squiggles, but these must be reduced to a very small size for this exercise. This is best achieved by importing your line drawings into a graphics program that allows for easy rescaling. Illustration by the author.

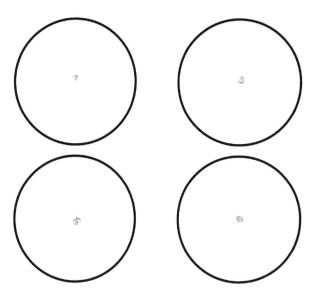

Figure 5.4 The drawings of Figure 5.3 reduced in size for students to attempt drawing. Illustration by the author.

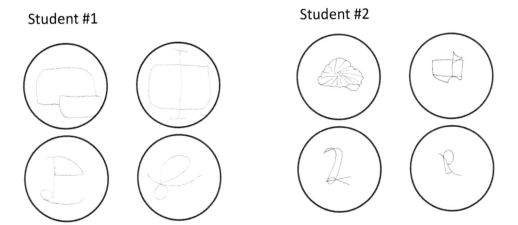

Figure 5.5 Examples of student drawings from my class using the tiny drawings in Figure 5.4. Again, there is emergent pragnanz in the form of symmetry, contour completion, and other "nicer" forms. Photo by the author.

they would look like if drawn much larger? As in the Telephone exercise, compare these magnified drawings to the original images and look for more goodness of form – more symmetry, more closed contours, more lines that meet at contours etc. In Figure 5.5 you can see some examples of things my students drew in response to the tiny figures pictured in Figure 5.4.

As in the Telephone game, this is another look at the heuristics the visual system is using to make guesses about visual forms given limited or uncertain data. Unlike our game of Telephone, you can also see some idiosyncrasies in terms of what kinds of forms different artists were willing to include in their own drawing. These two participants appear to differ a lot in terms of the complexity they were willing to include: The seashell shape at the upper left of the second group of images has a lot of interesting detail, for example. While it is challenging to really pin down what individual differences in these drawings might mean in terms of fundamentally different processes for perceptual organization, looking at lots of different drawings of the same tiny shapes across different participants makes it possible to see many variations on how pragnanz manifests itself under these circumstances. Experiment with different starting doodles and different kinds of irregularity to see what your observers' visual systems come up with when they can't just rely on a clear look at the shape.

Overall, both of these exercises demonstrate the range of Gestalt principles for perceptual organization and offer some intuition for what "good form" means to our visual system. The Gestalt psychologists' list of principles included the specific items I listed above (symmetry, uniformity) and several others. A guiding principle that is evident across nearly all of these is *similarity*: Visual elements that are similar to one another should be grouped together. Similarity can be defined in many ways, of course, including similarity of motion (which the Gestalt psychologists called "common fate"), similarity of position in the visual field (which the Gestalt psychologists called "grouping by proximity"), and similarity of shape or color. These different aspects of visual similarity all contribute to your own perceptual organization within a complex scene. Elements that are rather different in size may still be grouped together if they are similar enough in color and motion, for example. Elements that are very close together may be segmented separately from one another if their appearance is too different as well. In the next exercise, we will examine a particular kind of perceptual organization, amodal completion, as a means of exploring how specific aspects of similarity trade off against one another during the grouping of visual elements according to good form.

Illusory Volumes and Surfaces with Paper Inducers

One Gestalt principle that governs how perceptual organization manifests in some scenes is the principle of good continuation. To put it plainly, nearby edges that are aligned in terms of their relative position and their relative orientation are said to be *relatable*, meaning that they could be connected by a line that would not need to bend too sharply to accommodate the different tilts of the two small edges under consideration. Good continuation can lead edges in a simple scene to be grouped together into a larger unit, leading to the perception of a contour that extends between the edges that have been perceptually grouped. Because those contours are not actually present in the image, we refer to these as *subjective contours*. The phenomenon of subjective contours is a good one to explore further, especially given that we saw how cells in the primary visual cortex measured small lines and edges across the visual field at different orientations. The combination of those local measurements into something larger is a key contributing factor to our experience of these subjective edges following perceptual grouping.

Subjective contours are also a powerful demonstration of the visual system's capacity for perceptual organization and inference beyond raw image data. In the classic Kanizsa triangle, small inducing contours positioned in a manner that is consistent with the presence of an equilateral triangle lead to the perception of extended subjective contours and a distinct triangular surface when neither of these elements are objectively present in the image. In this exercise, we will use variations on the typical Kanizsa Pac-Men (Kanizsa, 1976) inducing edges as a means of testing the strength and limits of illusory contours. By making free-form subjective contours and shapes on paper, you will be able to examine the limits of good continuation and subsequent amodal competition of various shapes and contours (Figure 5.6).

Things you will need:

- Cut-out inducing elements (Pac-Man shapes and concave/convex spikes included in the Supplementary Material but also easy to make on your own).
- Scissors.
- A few images of different textures or scenes.

Illusory Contours and Shapes on a Uniform Background

Begin by cutting out the various Pac-Man inducers from the sheet of paper provided in the text after these instructions. You will see that there are a range of angles in each "Pac-Man" spanning acute, right, and obtuse angles. Try arranging them on a blank piece of paper to make a range of subjective shapes. Start with triangles, squares, and rectangles before moving on to more complex and free-form arrangements that may incorporate many different inducing elements (see Figure 5.7). As you make these shapes, you should be able to observe how subjective contours can be curved, straight, or even have corners within them in some circumstances (Figure 5.7).

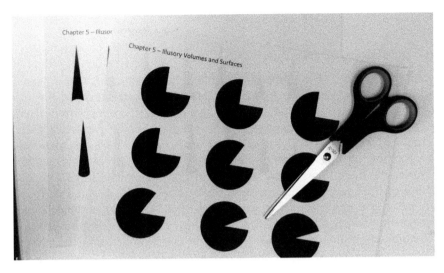

Figure 5.6 A sheet of inducing Pac-Man elements, spike elements, and scissors to cut these out with. Photo by the author.

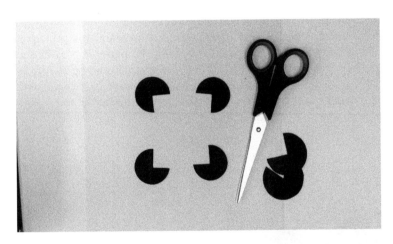

Figure 5.7 By placing the Pac-Man shapes on a blank background you can make a wide variety of illusory surfaces. Photo by the author.

Besides observing that one can obtain various shapes by arranging these differently on the page, you can also test the limits of illusory contour formation via good continuation. How far away can inducers be from one another before the subjective contour is no longer so vivid? Try turning neighboring inducing contours away from one another until the illusory contour or surface is broken. Likewise, try pulling the inducing elements away from one another on the page to see how far apart they can get before you begin to lose the impression that there is a subjective contour or surface. These are questions you can answer either intuitively by dragging and turning inducers until it feels like the shape is less coherent, or that you can explore quantitatively by making measurements of the distances and angles that are right at threshold for seeing the shape. Try to determine some specific limits to when small edges are relatable to one another so that amodal completion can be carried out.

Illusory Contours and Shapes on Complex Backgrounds

After you've determined some of the properties of the inducing elements that influence the strength of the subjective shapes you can form with these inducers, experiment with the background, too. Try placing the inducing elements on noise patterns with different properties (grainy noise vs. coarse, smoky noise) and on natural scenes. Personally, I find that natural scenes lead to an especially vivid subjective shape. These different background scenes have the potential to interfere with the inducing edges that are visible in the Pac-Man shapes. Again, are there limits to the strength of good continuation that depend on the appearance of the image around the edges we are hoping will be connected via a subjective contour? Try manipulating the contrast of the Pac-Man elements against your background image by printing them out in a fainter gray color, or using background images that have high-contrast edges of their own (Figure 5.8).

Illusory 3D Volumes with 2D Inducers

Your visual system is capable of making much more complex inferences about shape based on a small number of inducing contours spread out across space. Specifically, we can push your visual system out of the 2D plane and into 3D space using different inducers arranged to suggest various volumetric elements that arise from perceptual organization principles as well (Tse, 1998). Cut out the spiky inducing elements from the patterns provided in this section, and arrange these on the paper to make a subjective volumetric shape. In particular, you will notice that some of these small spikes have a concave base that curves inward, while others have a convex base that curves outward. Try arranging the spikes with

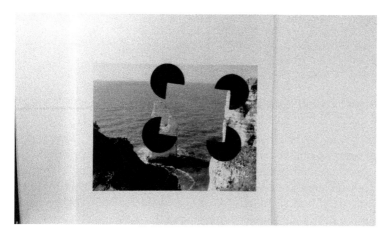

Figure 5.8 The strength of subjective contours varies as a function of the background region. Try different textures, colors, and scenes to see which ones lead to the strongest illusory shapes. Photo by the author.

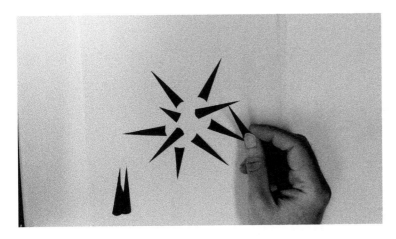

Figure 5.9 The spike elements can be used to create illusory volumes rather than planar illusory surfaces. Other kinds of inducing elements support volumetric percepts like this, so experiment with other shapes to see what works best. Photo by the author.

a concave base on the page so that the curved bases can be connected via good continuation to make some sort of rounded closed contour, like a sort of lumpy, puffy cloud. Next, try putting some spikes with a convex base in the interior of this cloud-like shape. This should allow you to make a variety of puffball shapes like the one in Figure 5.9 that you may be able to perceive as having 3D volume despite being made up solely of 2D elements. As with the 2D inducers, what are the limits of these subjective shapes? Are there other inducing elements that help support the perception of illusory volumes? In particular, try experimenting with the convexity or concavity of lots of different shapes to see what kinds of forms you can make. The various manipulations of distance between the inducing elements, relative orientation of the spikes, and other factors that might strengthen or weaken the good continuation between the curved parts of the shapes should have an impact here (Figure 5.9).

Freehand Neon Color Spreading

In both of the demonstrations of surface and volume completion we've covered so far, contours and corners were crucial to eliciting the perception of either a 2D or 3D shape that wasn't actually present in the image. In this exercise, you'll experiment with another completion phenomenon that depends critically on contrast and color relationships rather than contour: *Neon color spreading.* This phenomenon is particularly intriguing because, while the resulting illusory surfaces resemble those formed from Kanizsa-like inducing elements, the factors that influence the strength of this illusion are different than those that affect the surface completion phenomena you've already explored (Watanabe & Sato, 1989). This suggests that the way neon color spreading works is distinct from the way other illusory surfaces are formed, hinting at contributions for other visual processes that support inferences about properties like achromatic and chromatic contrast and transparency (Figure 5.10).

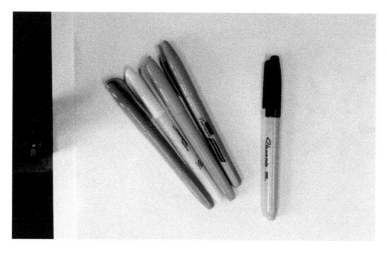

Figure 5.10 Markers in a range of colors, including neon highlighters, and a black marker should
       be all you need to create vivid neon color spreading phenomena. Photo by the author.

Things you will need:

- Blank paper.
- Neon highlighters and ordinary color markers.
- A sharpie or other black marker.

Neon color spreading depends on creating patterns of dark and colored lines that suggest
the presence of an illusory colored surface that the visual system then interpolates based
on the lines present in the image. Concentric circles turn out to be an excellent inducing
stimulus for this phenomenon, so begin by sketching nested rings (I'd suggest three rings
per bullseye pattern) arranged so that you have four sets of rings arranged in a square
configuration.

With these light pencil sketches in place, use one of your highlighters (blue is likely a
good color to start with) to trace the inner quarter of each bullseye pattern. That is, for
each of your four concentric ring patterns, color the arcs that face towards the other bullseyes using your highlighter. When you've finished this, trace the remaining arcs in all four
bullseye patterns using your black marker. When you're done, you should have something
like Figure 5.11, and I'd encourage you to make a few versions of this stimulus so that you
can try out your different colors. Hopefully, these will all yield a vivid percept of an illusory
square defined by the colored arcs (Figure 5.11).

Color and Contrast in Neon Color Spreading

Now that you have some successful examples of neon color spreading, it's time to see what
factors may strengthen or weaken this effect. Try making versions of this stimulus using
colored markers that are not neon colors: how does the strength of these illusory surfaces
compare to what you got with the neon markers? You might also try varying the contrast
between the colored parts of the arcs and the dark marker – what happens when you use a

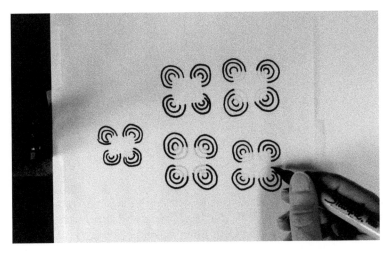

Figure 5.11 Example patterns that elicit neon color spreading. Note that the strength of the effect depends somewhat on the color of the interior patterns. Try different variations of these patterns to see when you obtain and don't obtain the effect. Photo by the author.

non-black marker for the outer parts of the arcs? What about drawing these same patterns on a sheet of gray paper instead of a white paper? You can also try viewing the patterns with sunglasses on to see how contrast affects the illusion.

Another interesting test of how the phenomenon works is to try doing the whole thing in grayscale without using color at all. In this version of the illusion, try making the inner arcs light gray and the outer arcs dark. Now flip this arrangement to make the inner arcs darker and the outer arcs lighter gray. An interesting observation about these two stimuli is that only one of them (the one with darker arcs on the inside) is consistent with an interpretation of the stimulus in terms of transparency (a translucent sheet of gray film placed on top of light gray bullseyes would make the inner arcs dark): Which stimulus appears to yield the strongest illusory surface? What does this tell you about the role of transparency estimates in this effect? As I mentioned at the beginning of this chapter, your visual system uses a range of different heuristics to group, segment, and otherwise organize the information provided by early stages of visual processing. Simple completion effects like these provide a useful mini-laboratory for testing the boundaries of those heuristics and refining your understanding of what the rules for organizing your vision appear to be.

References

Kanizsa, G. (1976). Subjective contours. *Scientific American, 234*(4), 48–52. https://doi.org/10.1038/scientificamerican0476-48

Metzger, W. (2009). *Laws of seeing*. MIT Press.

Tse, P. U. (1998). Illusory volumes from conformation. *Perception, 27*(8), 977–992. https://doi.org/10.1068/p270977

Watanabe, T., & Sato, T. (1989). Effects of luminance contrast on color spreading and illusory contour in the neon color spreading effect. *Perception & Psychophysics, 45*(5), 427–430. https://doi.org/10.3758/bf03210716

6 Brightness and Color Constancy

In our previous discussion of the way the retina works, we talked about how the photoreceptors transduce incoming light to provide the visual system with measurements of both the intensity of light and the wavelengths of light that are present in different parts of the visual field. These first steps towards measuring light intensity and color are not the final word on our experience of both brightness and color, however. Our subjective experience of light-dark intensity and color begin with the retina, but also depend on cortical processing at later stages of visual processing too.

In particular, cortical processing of brightness and color supports *perceptual constancy* with regard to these properties of visual scenes. This term refers to the estimation of stable properties of the environment despite variability in the measurements we obtain from the environment itself. In general, one important feature of the visual system beyond the early stages of processing that we have already covered is to use measurements of visual structure as the basis for estimating environmental properties. These kinds of problems are often referred to as *inverse problems* because the goal is to start with some set of measurements and work backwards to the causes of that data. Inverse problems tend to be difficult to solve because they are frequently *underconstrained*. This term refers to a situation in which we lack enough data to come up with an unambiguous best answer concerning the problem we are trying to solve.

To understand what all of this means with regard to brightness and color perception, it's important to note that the light that ends up landing on the retina depends on two properties of the visual scene itself: (1) The light that is illuminating the objects and surfaces we are looking at, and (2) The proportion of that light that the object or surface reflects towards our eye. Though illumination can vary depending on the time of day (our **Observing Color Change in a Day** exercise demonstrates this) or the type of artificial light we are using in an indoor setting, the reflectance properties of objects and surfaces do not change so readily. This means that, though an object or surface may look different moment to moment depending on the light that is shining on it, our visual system might be able to solve this particular inverse problem to provide us with a stable response that reflects the color something *is* rather than the color that it looks like now. The trick is finding a way to start with the raw data provided by the photoreceptors and using that as the basis for inferring the illumination and the reflectance that produced it. This inference depends on more complex processing that is downstream from early visual stages. In these exercises, our goal is to explore the nature and limitations of these computations using **Simultaneous Brightness and Color Contrast** as a demonstration of how profoundly these computations can change our perception of objects and surfaces and examining the **Spatial Scale in Color Constancy** computations.

DOI: 10.4324/9781032691169-7

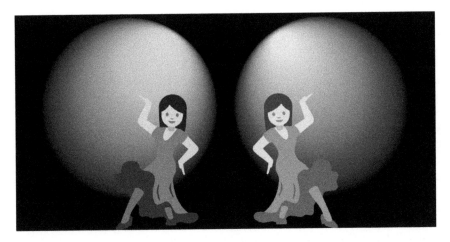

Figure 6.1 The light that reaches our eye from an object or a surface is a combination of the illuminating light source's ingredients and the proportion of those ingredients that are reflected by the object or surface. This means that different illumination conditions can lead to very different light spectra reaching our eye even though the objects and surfaces do not change. In this cartoon, the dancer's dress and skin tone are not actually becoming more yellow or more blue but are instead being illuminated by a spotlight that changes color. Image credit: cmglee, Google, CC BY-SA 4.0 <https://creativecommons.org/licenses/by-sa/4.0>, via Wikimedia Commons.

Observing Color Change in a Day

So far, we've talked about measuring the wavelengths present in different parts of the visual field using the photoreceptors (the cones in particular) and the color-sensitive cells in the LGN and V1. One feature of the light that arrives at the eye, however, is that it is actually a product of two things in the environment. First, the light that arrives at your eye from an object or surface depends on the light that is illuminating the scene: A reddish light shining on an object will lead to a different outcome than a bluish light shining on it. Second, the object or surface itself will only reflect some proportion of light at each wavelength, further influencing the light that will make it to the observer. While the *reflectance* of objects or surfaces tends not to change, the *illumination* of those items may vary (Figure 6.1). In this exercise, you will observe that variability by taking pictures of the same scene at different times of day.

Things you will need:

- A camera.
- A piece of cardstock with a hole punched into it.

The procedure here is quite simple: Choose an outdoor scene that has a variety of colors in it (it is especially useful to get something close to white or off-white in the mix) and take three pictures of the same scene: (1) Early in the morning, while the sun is relatively low, (2) At midday while the sun is high in the sky, and (3) At dusk as the sun is setting. If you like, you might also try using a scene that includes streetlights and other artificial lights that are only turned on for part of the day. These different conditions involve varying illumination due to the sun passing through more or less of the atmosphere at different times of day, or due to the presence of any artificial lights you may have in your scene. While the illumination changes, however, the reflectance of the objects or surfaces does not change – what consequence does this have on your perception of the color of those items?

Take a look at the same portion of the scene (say a part of a white wall or a section of the road) in each of your three images. How different would you say that the color of this item is across your three images? Now, look at the same region through the hole you have punched in your cardstock – set the card on the image so you are covering up everything around the target region, but the color is visible through the punched hole. You should see that the color looks quite different across the three images.

We'll revisit these ideas in the **Spatial Scale in Color Constancy** exercise, but for now the big idea is to take this as an important fact regarding natural scenes: The color of the light reflecting off of an object or surface may vary by quite a lot, but it would be nice for our vision to be capable of understanding that there is something about the object that is also staying stable. That perception of stability is called *color constancy* or *brightness constancy* and is part of a larger goal more broadly referred to as *perceptual constancy*. This latter term refers to more generally achieving the perception of stable properties of the environment despite variability in the appearance of the environment.

Simultaneous Brightness and Color Contrast

Our perception of how bright parts of a scene are and the color of the objects and surfaces in a scene each begin with physical properties of a light wave (the amplitude and wavelength, respectively) and the photoreceptors' responses to those. Because these are the starting point for your visual system's attempts to infer illumination and reflectance from the neural signal, the same physical stimulus can look remarkably different under different circumstances. Here, you will examine some contextual effects on color appearance induced by brightness and color gradients printed on paper. The big idea here is that brightness and color are not just things we measure but are instead things that we estimate. The malleability of our subjective experience of the same stimulus demonstrates the impact of downstream cortical processes on brightness and color perception (Figure 6.2).

Things you will need:

- Print-outs of color and luminance gradients and a few luminance gratings. (See the Supplementary Materials for images you can use.)
- Scissors.

Simultaneous Brightness Contrast on a Black/White Gradient

We'll begin by seeing how the appearance of an object that has stable reflectance properties can nonetheless change depending on the context that the object appears in. Using the grayscale gradient included in the Supplementary Material, cut out the small gray square in the corner and confirm that it is roughly the same gray value as the very center of the large rectangle. If you want to be extra certain about this, you can even print a second copy of the rectangle and cut out a small square from the middle of the pattern to use with the intact gradient. In any event, hold it in the middle to confirm that it looks medium gray to you.

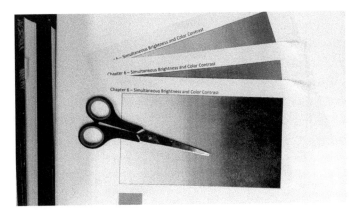

Figure 6.2 Brightness and color gradients, square probe patches, and scissors to cut these patterns out. Photo by the author.

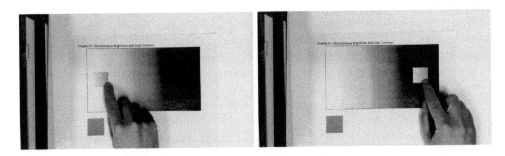

Figure 6.3 The same probe patch varies substantially in how light or dark it appears as you move it to different parts of the intensity gradient. Photo by the author.

Continue by moving the square left to right across the middle of the black/white gradient. Though the piece of paper you're sliding is obviously not changing, you should see a big change in how bright it appears to be. At left, the square should look to be very light gray, while at right it should look much darker. The images in Figure 6.3 capture some of this effect but setting it in motion for yourself is much more dramatic – and tends to impress people if you want to show off! (Figure 6.3).

Simultaneous Color Contrast (and Maybe Brightness Too?)

Repeat these steps with the different color gradients included here too. Each one comes with a square taken from the middle of the pattern, which should shift in hue as you move it from left to right. In Figure 6.4, you can maybe see that the square looks a little greener (and maybe darker) on the left and a little redder (and maybe brighter) on the right (Figure 6.4).

Now that you have all these little squares cut out, swap them around across the different gradients to see what happens when different colors and brightness move around

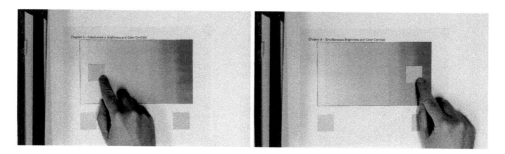

Figure 6.4 The apparent color of a probe patch can also be made to vary by moving it across a color gradient. Photo by the author.

on different backgrounds. How does the light/dark context affect the squares printed in color? How do different color gradients affect matched vs. mismatched color objects or objects in grayscale? Can you make some color appear in a gray object by surrounding it with color?

The main conclusion I want you to draw from these demonstrations is that brightness and color are estimated from parts of an image in a way that must depend on the context that an object or surface appears in. Note especially that, compared to our examples of objects appearing different under different illumination conditions, these effects only depend on the color and grayscale values that surround the small square we are moving around. These demonstrations show that the surrounding brightness or hue of an image region can have a large influence on what an object in that region looks like, turning objects different colors or gray values even when objective measurements of light coming from the object's surface wouldn't vary at all. To put it another way, a photometer that measured the light coming from our small squares would always say the same thing, but your visual system delivers very different experiences of these small squares depending on where you place them on these gradient backgrounds. This means that your visual system must be doing something more than a photometer does, and I've suggested in the introduction to this section that it's doing this in service of *perceptual constancy* for brightness and color. What exactly is it doing, however? Can we say anything about the nature of this process to help us understand how it works? This simple illusion still presents a number of interesting questions for the field of vision science, and relatively recent work has explored the stages of visual processing at which it appears to result (Sinha et al., 2020). In our next exercise, we will make some observations of our own using manipulated images to try and understand some intuitive parameters of how your visual system tries to estimate object and surface reflectance from raw image data.

Spatial Scale in Color Constancy

The previous exercise (**Simultaneous Brightness and Color Contrast**) demonstrated that context can affect perceived brightness and color profoundly. This raises both the question of "How?" and the question of "Why?" One way to answer the second question is to appeal to the value of color constancy – the ability to measure the color of light reflected by an object despite changes in the illuminating light. The wavelength information that reaches the retina from a surface is a combination of the contents of

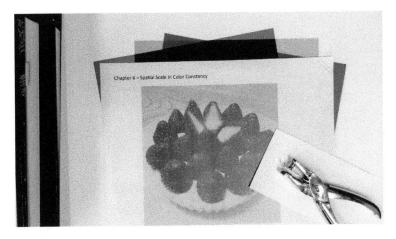

Figure 6.5 Akiyoshi Kitaoka's "No Red Pixel Strawberries" image is a wonderful starting point for examining the limits of color constancy in complex images. We will use this image, some color gels, and a piece of cardstock with a small hole punched into it as well. Photo by the author.

the illumination and the reflectance properties of the surface itself. While the former can change, the latter is more likely to be stable. Obtaining that stable measurement depends on using context in some way to come up with a guess about object or surface reflectance. In this exercise, we'll examine some manipulated images to accomplish two things. First, we'll confirm that your visual system really is delivering a stable appearance of object and surface reflectance via these downstream cortical processes that incorporate scene context into brightness and color perception. Second, we'll examine how much context the visual system appears to use to accomplish this feat. While we won't fully describe the process by which reflectance is inferred from earlier measurements of light intensity and wavelength, we will determine some constraints on how that process appears to work in complex images (Figure 6.5).

Things you will need:

- Some specific images: Akiyoshi Kitaoka's "No Red Pixel Strawberries," a colorful natural scene, and a Mondrian pattern. (See the Supplementary Materials for images you can use.)
- Color gels (or color transparency film if you prefer) of different colors (red, green, blue).
- A small piece of cardstock with a hole punched into it.

What Color Are Those Strawberries Really?

Begin by inspecting the strawberries depicted in Kitaoka's image of strawberries. Though you can probably see something is a little odd in this picture, I also imagine that they look fairly red to you. Choose the part of the image that looks the reddest and match the color that you see either with a digital color picker (like an RGB slider) or by choosing crayons or colored pencils that provide an approximate match to your experience (Figure 6.6).

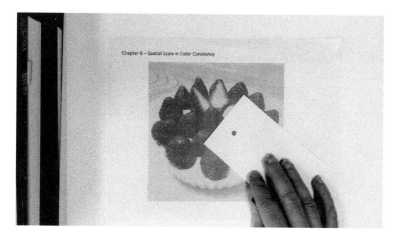

Figure 6.6 First, match the apparent color of the strawberries as you experience them in the full image. This will probably be a reddish color. Then, if you restrict your view of the strawberries to a very small patch, you should find that the apparent red color yields to a blue-green-gray color. Photo by the author.

Continue by placing the piece of cardstock over the image so that the small hole you punched into it is over the part of the image you selected as the reddest area. As you look at this same part of the picture through this little window, what color and brightness do you see? Once again, use either a digital color picker or a set of crayons or colored pencils to match your experience as closely as you can. My guess is that while you probably picked a reddish shade the first time you looked at the picture, you probably decided that a sort of gray-green color was a better match when you looked at the same region through the aperture.

There are two important points here I want to emphasize. First, let's give our visual system credit for accomplishing something rather remarkable: Despite the fact that the image has no truly red pixels in it, whatever your downstream color processing is doing resulted in you seeing these strawberries as fairly red. This is important support for the statements I made in our introduction – downstream processing of color and brightness helps us achieve perceptual constancy. Though these objects aren't reflecting light with long wavelengths towards your eye very much at all, your visual system is able to work out that the strawberries would reflect more long wavelength light than anything else. That estimation of how these objects would reflect different wavelengths of light results in your subjective experience of the strawberries as reddish in color. The second point we should dwell on for a moment is what changed when you looked at the reddest part of the image through the aperture. The fact that your experience of a red strawberry vanished and was replaced by an experience of seeing a gray-green patch of image demonstrates that the computations for inferring object and surface reflectance depend on seeing local context around the target image region. By limiting the field of view with the cardboard aperture, you also limited the visual system's ability to adjust the raw wavelength informa-tion reflecting from the page to arrive at a red percept. Together these outcomes dem-onstrate that some of the work being done to arrive at your experience of redness in this case depends on processing this picture at the appropriate (fairly large) spatial scale and finding some way to undo the compression of color values we've imposed on the image (Shapiro et al., 2018).

You can try estimating how much local context is needed for this process to work by applying holes that are increasingly large to your cardstock until the red percept returns. Try this out to see if you and other observers consistently identify an area of roughly the same size.

Make Your Own "No-Red-Pixels" Image (and Test It)

The "no-red-pixels" strawberries were created using a technique called histogram compression, but we can use analog tools to make our own version of these images. Select a natural image with many different bright colors in it and place one of your colored gels over top of it. Even with this color gel changing the wavelength information that is getting to your retina dramatically, you likely still see a good range of different colors in your picture, including some reds, yellows, and blues. Experiment with different color gels to see which ones support color constancy and which ones do not – green tends to be especially good, but red tends to be poor. Also, repeat the exercises we described above with the cardstock and the small aperture as before to determine how much context is needed to achieve color constancy with your image (Figure 6.7).

Using "Mondrians" to Test the Role of Object Knowledge on Color Constancy

Image context of some amount is clearly important for achieving color and brightness constancy, but how and why? Here are two ideas about how this might work that we'll test in one more set of observations. One idea is that your visual system uses the measurements

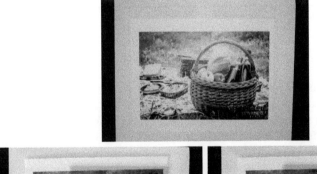

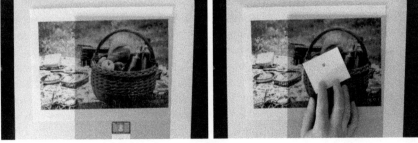

Figure 6.7 You can make your version of the "No Red Pixel Strawberries" image by placing your color gels (one at a time) on top of a colorful natural image. Photo by the author.

of intensity and wavelength content collected over some portion of the image to come up with a correction for those values based solely on the numbers appearing in that image region. If the region that we're looking at is too small, maybe there just aren't enough numbers to calculate the things we need for that correction to do much to the picture. Here is another idea that is a little more complicated, though: Maybe what your visual system is really doing is trying to recognize the objects and surfaces you are looking at so that you can use your knowledge of color-object joint statistics to guide your inferences about reflectance properties of the things you see. For example, if you can recognize that the objects in our first image are in fact strawberries, that label is a strong clue that they ought to be red. Likewise, if you're able to recognize the grassy textures in the picnic scene or the loaf of bread in the basket, this might allow your visual system to rely on what you know about grass tending to be green and bread tending to be sort of golden-brown. In this case, the amount of local context might be important because seeing too little of a scene makes it much more difficult to recognize the objects and textures we are looking at.

We'll test these two ideas by using an image called a "Mondrian" that has no recognizable objects in it. Instead, this image is made up of overlapping geometric shapes, like rectangles and circles, that are each a different color. Your visual system shouldn't have too many strong biases to think that a particular rectangle or circle should be yellow or blue most of the time, so these images remove the possibility that color constancy depends on object or surface recognition. If we find that you're able to achieve color constancy in these images, that would be a strong hint that this process doesn't rely much on recognizing objects, so you know what color they ought to be. On the other hand, if we aren't able to achieve color constancy in this case, that would be a strong hint that we do need those recognition processes to help us infer reflectance from raw measurements of incoming light (Figure 6.8).

Repeat the steps described above for our natural images with the gel and the cardstock applied to the Mondrian image. You should see that the same effects are easily obtainable, suggesting that we don't need to recognize objects or surfaces to estimate their reflectance. Instead, there is some computation that must operate just on the photoreceptor values in the image array without requiring us to understand the identity of the objects and textures we're seeing.

These demonstrations help us understand some of the limits of color constancy in terms of the amount of image context that's needed to achieve it and the "illuminant" conditions that do and don't support robust estimates of object reflectance. Multiple algorithms have been proposed to account for the human visual system's color constancy abilities. The most widely taught of these is Edwin Land's Retinex algorithm (see McCann et al., 1976 for a discussion of the application of Retinex to Mondrian patterns like those above), which uses assumptions about the nature of illumination and reflectance gradients to separate these components of an image from one another. Though beyond the scope of this textbook, this algorithm is an example of the kind of computation that can lead to a robust inference of object and surface reflectance without the need to recognize objects and textures first. We should note, however, that these processes don't always work perfectly, which can lead to fascinating phenomena like "#TheDress" – a blue-black dress that was depicted in a photograph in such a way that it looked white-gold to some people, blue-black to others, and made everyone terribly angry and confused for a while in the late 2010's (Dixon & Shapiro, 2017).

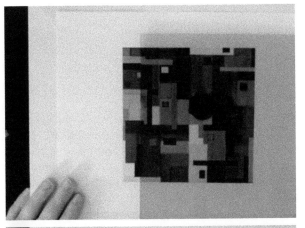

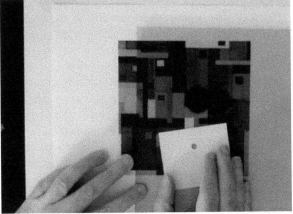

Figure 6.8 Does our color constancy depend on knowing color-object associations? We can examine
this with random "Mondrian" patterns that vary in color but are not at all recognizable
objects. Photo by the author.

The Role of Edges in Interpreting Illumination and Reflectance

We've seen in the previous exercises that your perception of the brightness and color
of different parts of a complex scene depends on how your visual system attributes the
way illumination and reflectance both contribute to the appearance of each image patch.
Working with the "No Red Pixel Strawberries" image and related manipulations of global
brightness and color appearance, we could see that your visual system does some kind of
work over larger spatial scales to estimate reflectance and achieve color constancy. In this
exercise, we'll use a simple demonstration to show how your visual system also uses image
gradients (also known as edges) where there is a transition between light and dark to make
estimates of the contribution of illumination and reflectance to the appearance of image
regions. While we aren't going to completely specify how these aspects of image appearance are used quantitatively to come up with specific estimates of image illumination and
reflectance, these demonstrations should give you a sense of the kinds of heuristics your
visual system uses to come up with these guesses about the visual environment.

Things you will need:

- A flashlight or other relatively small light source with a small beam.
- A piece of cardstock or other stiff, opaque material.
- A dark marker.
- A light background to draw on.

We'll begin by using our light source and the piece of cardstock that we have to cast the shadow of some simple shape onto our light background. Cut a random shape out of your cardstock and try to either suspend it from somewhere or attach it to some kind of stand (I used a twisted paperclip and a base made from binder clips and a pencil in Figure 6.9) so that you can shine your flashlight behind it, casting a shadow on the paper. As you do so, take a look at the edge of this shadow. My guess is that even though the shadow will be fairly dark, the very edge of the shadow will be somewhat "fuzzy" and not as sharp as a line you might draw with ink or marker (Figure 6.9).

Another simple observation to make about this shadow is something so fundamental that it's easy to overlook: This dark spot on the paper looks like an illumination change to you, not a reflectance change! That is, shadows look like shadows – they don't look like the paper itself actually changes from light to dark. This implies that your visual system is making an estimate of how illumination and reflectance each contribute to the appearance of the surface across the page, leading to the perception of that dark spot as an illumination variation rather than a reflectance variation. How does it do this? One piece of this estimate has to do with the fuzzy nature of the shadow boundary – because light sources tend to have a finite extent to them, shadows tend to have fuzzy boundaries as light from different parts of the source can find slightly different paths around the external contour of the 3D shape on their way to the surface where the shadow is cast. This means that your visual system can try to work backwards using the characteristics of the edges that it is presented with to determine where changes in brightness or color are the result of illumination or reflectance: A blurry edge probably means a change of illumination, while a very sharp edge probably means a change in reflectance. To test this idea, we'll change our shadow's

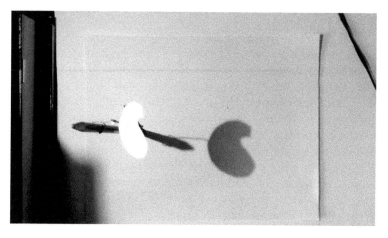

Figure 6.9 A cast shadow on a piece of paper has a fuzzy boundary. Photo by the author.

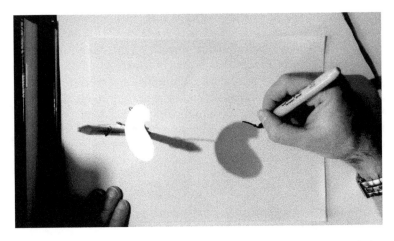

Figure 6.10 Trace the external contour of your shadow using a very dark marker. Here, you can see I've traced the inner boundary as well, but you can trace as much or as little as you like. Photo by the author.

edge with our dark marker. Specifically, make that edge sharp by tracing the shadow's edge with a thick, very dark marker line (Figure 6.10).

What I hope you can see after doing this is that the shadow looks less like an illumination change and much more like a bit of dark paint on the page. The sharpness of the boundary indeed appears to signal to your visual system that there is a potential change in reflectance here rather than a change in illumination, which leads the same gray value inside the shadow to be attributed to the surface rather than to the light source (Figure 6.11).

It's worth taking a look back at our demonstrations of **Simultaneous Brightness and Color Contrast** up above with these ideas in mind. This is also an interesting starting

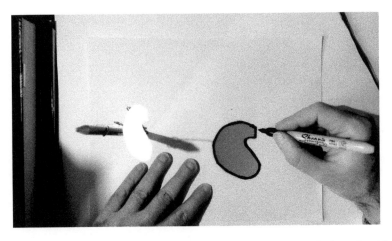

Figure 6.11 Adding a dark boundary to the edge of your shadow should make this illumination change look much more like a change in reflectance. That is, your shadow should look more like paint. Photo by the author.

point for some ecological study of how different kinds of edges work in the natural world to see how frequently this heuristic we've played with is actually true and how often it is violated. When it is violated, does your visual system still come up with a percept that reflects the true state of the world? Like most inference problems, perfection is probably too much to expect and the places where the process breaks down are some of the most informative pieces of evidence about how the underlying mechanisms work to support your visual experience. Keep these ideas in mind as we continue to explore other kinds of inverse problem that your visual system needs to solve in the next two chapters, each concerned with a different property of the environment that we would like our visual system to estimate from images.

References

Dixon, E. L., & Shapiro, A. G. (2017). Spatial filtering, color constancy, and the color-changing dress. *Journal of Vision*, *17*(3), 7. https://doi.org/10.1167/17.3.7

McCann, J. J., McKee, S. P., & Taylor, T. H. (1976). Quantitative studies in retinex theory. A comparison between theoretical predictions and observer responses to the "color mondrian" experiments. *Vision Research*, *16*(5), 445–458. https://doi.org/10.1016/0042-6989(76)90020-1

Shapiro, A., Hedjar, L., Dixon, E., & Kitaoka, A. (2018). Kitaoka's tomato: Two simple explanations based on information in the stimulus. *i-Perception*, *9*(1), 2041669517749601. https://doi.org/10.1177/2041669517749601

Sinha, P., Crucilla, S., Gandhi, T., Rose, D., Singh, A., Ganesh, S., Mathur, U., & Bex, P. (2020). Mechanisms underlying simultaneous brightness contrast: Early and innate. *Vision Research*, *173*, 41–49. https://doi.org/10.1016/j.visres.2020.04.012

7 Depth Perception

Besides recovering brightness and color from the measurements provided by early stages of visual processing, our visual system also estimates a number of other complex properties based on the limited data provided by the retina, the LGN, and V1. Here, we examine a particularly interesting problem: How do you get 3D information about the world back when you start by measuring light with a 2D retina? There are a range of *monocular depth cues* that are available to help us estimate depth with just one retinal image, and different *binocular depth cues* that are available if we can use both retinal images. Both types of cues to depth require that we make some critical assumptions about how 3D scenes are projected onto the 2D surfaces of the retinae, which we will explore in these exercises. First, we will examine linear perspective (a powerful monocular depth cue) in three exercises (**Ames Room**, **Ames Window**, and **Linear Perspective and Perceived Size/Depth**) to see how assumed relationships between 2D and 3D geometry can lead to dramatic distortions of perceived size and motion. Next, we will move on to the nature of binocular depth perception. First, we measure the extent of **Binocular Vergence** as a depth cue, followed by tutorials in how to make 3D images using **Red/Green Anaglyphs**, **Stereo Photography**, and **Random-Dot Stereograms**, all of which are useful tools for seeing how *binocular disparity* can be used to estimate depth from two retinal images (Figure 7.1).

Build a Model Ames Room

One of the most powerful ways to see how your visual system uses assumptions about the relationship between 3D scenes and 2D images is the Ames Room (Ames, 1952). This is a distorted room that looks like an ordinary rectangular space when viewed from a particular point in space, but is in fact shaped quite differently. Because of the assumptions that your visual system makes about depth based on the presumed shape of the room, objects placed in the Ames Room appear to change size in strange ways as they move around within it. The best way to see how and why this works is to build one yourself (Figure 7.2).

Things you will need:

- A printable Ames Room template (preferably on cardstock, but paper will do). See www.rigb.org/sites/default/files/attachments/ames_room_template_experimental_0 .pdf. There are others out there that are easy to find online, but this one is my favorite.
- Scissors.
- Cellophane tape.
- Some small figures or objects – LEGO minifigs or dollhouse objects work well.

DOI: 10.4324/9781032691169-8

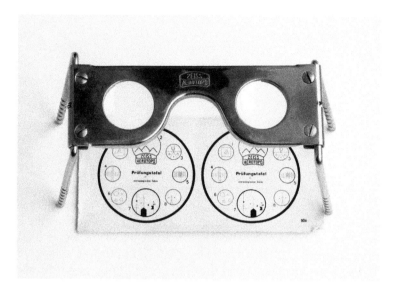

Figure 7.1 Understanding how image properties signal depth relationships makes it possible to create 3D experiences out of 2D images. These techniques have been used for nearly two centuries to make compelling stereoscopic images with viewers like this one. Joaquim Alves Gaspar, CC BY-SA 3.0 <http://creativecommons.org/licenses/by-sa/3.0/>, via Wikimedia Commons.

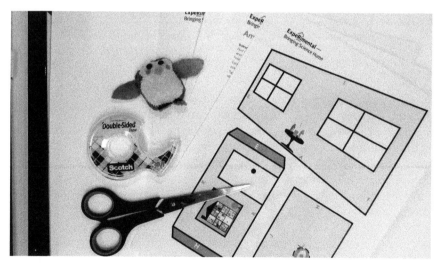

Figure 7.2 A model Ames Room template, some scissors and tape to assemble it, and a small object to place inside of it. Photo by the author.

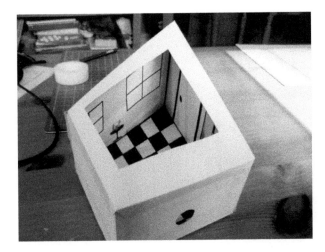

Figure 7.3 The assembled Ames Room has an odd 3D geometry when viewed from the outside, but it looks much more like a regular cube when viewed through the portal at the front of the room. Photo by the author.

Build the Model Room

The first thing we need to do is actually construct the model Ames Room out of paper or (preferably) something like cardstock. Either material will work, but be careful to crease everything very sharply if you're using a flimsier material. Once you have the room assembled, take note of the true dimensions of the room. You may have found that the assembly could be a little tricky due to the fact that the walls of the room are shaped quite differently than a typical dollhouse room. This is because the specific geometry of the Ames Room is designed to achieve visual effects that are a consequence of the visual system's assumptions about the space that the walls of the room take up. Begin by looking at the different shapes depicted on the walls and floor of the room from some different viewpoints to see how these shapes look different to you from different directions. These changes are all directly related to how the 3D position of these contours projects onto the 2D surface of your retina. If you like, it might be worth taking another look at the pinhole camera you made in earlier exercises to see how different 3D edges in the environment turn into 2D edges on the viewing screen of your pinhole camera (Figure 7.3).

Viewing Objects in the Room

Once the room is assembled, look at the rear wall through the viewing portal in the front. By looking through this portal, we are giving ourselves a specific 2D projection of this 3D shape to work with. Despite the fact that the back wall of the room is actually tilted rather sharply in depth, slanting away from you from the left side of the room to the right, the particular lines making up the four sides of the rear wall have been selected so that they project to the shape of a rectangle from this view. Likewise, though the checkerboard pattern on the floor is made up of different quadrilaterals that are not square at all, from this vantage point the floor should look like it has a regular pattern made up of squares. All of

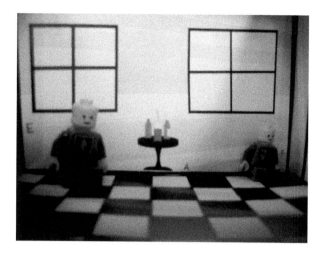

Figure 7.4 The inferred depth of the back wall, which appears flat but actually recedes in depth from left to right, leads to a profound size illusion when objects are placed in the back corners of the room. Photo by the author.

these features of the 2D appearance of the room are consistent with a 3D interpretation of the scene: This room looks like a simple 3D cube rather than the distorted shape we know we have built! This assumption leads your visual system to assume that the different sides of the back wall are at equal depth from you, so objects placed in the two corners can only look the way they do (one taking up far less space on the retina) because they are different sizes! This is why the LEGO figures you see here look like a large one and a small one rather than a near one and a far one (Figure 7.4).

Photographs of the Ames Room?

An important caveat remains, however. You probably can see in my photograph that there are a number of cues that give away the true state of things, and it's worth taking a moment to identify these reasons that the apparent size illusion between the two minifigs is not so strong in this picture compared to during direct viewing. In particular, the different amounts of blur in the image turn out to be an important monocular depth cue: Objects that differ in apparent blur probably differ in depth as well. In this photograph, this helps disambiguate the situation a little bit and weakens the size illusion induced by the room's shape. You can also see that the minifigs in Figure 7.4 don't take up the same space on the floor, which is evident from the checkerboard pattern: The left figure covers up a full row of this pattern, but the right one fits comfortably within about half a square. The basic illusion works, but these little disruptions of the effect also highlight that there are multiple monocular cues to depth that all contribute to your overall estimates of where things are in space. It is also the case that viewing the Ames Room with two eyes (binocular viewing) rather than just one will weaken the illusory effect (Pilewski & Martin, 1991). This also highlights how your perception of depth results from the combination of multiple cues.

Still, what is the basis for this powerful illusion when we are looking at the room itself rather than a photograph of it? This model leverages our visual system's use of the laws of *linear perspective* to manipulate our perception of size. Linear perspective refers to the lawful relationship between 3D contours and textures in the environment and the arrangement of these elements when they are projected onto a 2D surface. As a direct consequence of such a projection, certain 2D features of images indicate specific aspects of 3D layout. In particular, you may have heard of something called a *vanishing point*, which refers to a spot in 2D images of 3D scenes where lines that recede in depth away from the viewer in the environment meet in the 2D projection. Because this 3D layout (lines receding in depth) leads to a specific 2D structure (lines converging onto a point), your visual system can attempt to start from the 2D structure on the retina to work backwards to estimates of depth. In the Ames Room, this is primarily what is happening: The converging lines of the checkerboard floor, combined with the parallel edges of the back wall, all indicate a cube-like 3D layout. Your visual system is making assumptions about the relationship between 2D and 3D appearance that are right nearly all of the time, but we've carefully built this model room so that they are precisely wrong from the viewpoint we've chosen.

The Ames Room is a great deal of fun to play with. In particular, moving objects along the back wall while you or a friend watch through the peephole is a fun way to watch the perceived size of the object in the room change while it moves. Despite the fact that this is really an object looming towards you, it is very difficult to not see as an object that is growing as it slides instead. With your model room in hand, experiment with other object configurations and movements to see what things you observe as objects move within a space with a much different geometry than it appears to have.

Depth/Motion Confusion via the Ames Window

The Ames Room provides a nice demonstration of how miscalibrated estimates about depth can lead to misperceptions of size that are dramatic. The Ames Window (Gregory, 2009) relies on the same linear perspective cues to provide another set of depth estimates that turn out to be inaccurate, which then disrupt the perceived motion of the window. Together, these illusions reveal how strong geometric cues of depth can be and how competition between cues can play out as a function of uncertainty and salience (Figure 7.5).

Things you will need:

- An image of the Ames Window (see Supplementary Materials).
- String or a stick.
- Scissors.

Cut out two copies of the Ames Window pattern including the interior trapezoids. Using either some string, a stick, or, in Figure 7.5, some re-purposed rubber bands so that you have a means of allowing the window to spin left-to-right while held horizontally. Looking at it with both eyes open should look fine so long as you hold the window about 1–2 feet from your eyes, but closing one eye should lead the motion to be disrupted. Specifically, you may experience a sort of windshield-wiper effect where the window appears to rock back and forth rather than spin fully around. The trapezoid shape suggests that the smaller edge is further away from you than the larger one, leading to an estimate of motion that

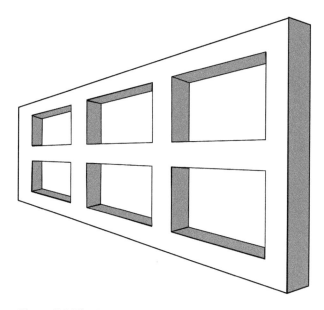

Figure 7.5 The Ames Window also depends on linear perspective cues for depth perception but leads to a disruption of motion perception rather than distorted size perception. VanBuren, CC BY-SA 3.0 <https://creativecommons.org/licenses/by-sa/3.0>, via Wikimedia Commons.

is based on a wrong assumption. Play with the speed of spinning to see how this affects this percept. You may also try looking at the Ames Window from further away (7–8 feet perhaps) with both of your eyes open.

Like the Ames Room, we have another object in which we have selected 2D features carefully to imply a specific 3D layout. In this case, the tilted lines of the Ames Window converge at a common vanishing point, which suggests that these are lines that recede in depth in the 3D scene. Of course, because they are really parallel to the plane of your eyes, this means that the change in appearance we observe as the Ames Window rotates is not the same as what we should expect if the left and right vertical edges were really at differ-ent depths. Besides providing another example of the strength of linear perspective cues for depth perception, this illusion shows us how assumptions about depth can interfere with other aspects of perception, including the size of objects in the Ames Room and the movement of objects in the Ames Window. The perspective cues in the Ames Window are also sufficiently powerful that they can even induce illusory proprioceptive sensations: Holding a model Ames Window that is a bit larger than this one with outstretched arms can make it feel like one of your hands is further away from you than the other (Bruno et al., 2006)! Depth estimates thus ultimately inform a range of other perceptual computa-tions and subjective experiences.

Linear Perspective and Perceived Size/Depth

Both the Ames Room and the Ames Window demonstrate how linear perspective can be used by the visual system to estimate depth in 3D scenes, leading to misperceptions of

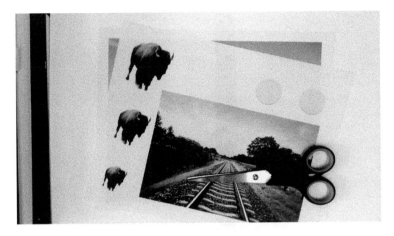

Figure 7.6 Images with strong perspective cues can also be used to induce size illusions. Photo by
the author.

size and motion. Here, you will explore size illusions induced by different aspects of scene
geometry to investigate how different 2D features are used to make guesses about scene
layout that ultimately lead to depth and size errors. Specifically, we will work with images
that have varying numbers of *vanishing points*, which refer to locations in the 2D image
where lines receding in depth in the environment converge (Figure 7.6).

Things you will need:

- Images of empty scenes with zero-, single-, and two-point perspective geometry. You
  can see my examples in the figures, but I'd suggest finding some favorites of your
  own.
- Some flat objects (cut-out shapes, stickers, or coins, e.g.) to move around on the images.
- Scissors.

All of these images depict 3D scenes with fairly simple geometry: A ground plane that
recedes in depth away from the viewer, with the addition of some vertical walls in the case
of our two-point perspective image. Despite the simplicity of these scenes, they all include
enough information to use assumptions about vanishing points and projective relationships between 3D scenes and 2D images to support estimates of depth based on what's visible in the image. In each case, we're going to use these 2D images to manipulate how we
perceive the size of 2D objects. Compared to our demonstrations with the Ames Window
and the Ames Room, these illusions highlight how much your visual system tries to do
solely with 2D information, leading to illusory percepts that don't require us to carefully
manipulate 3D structure in the environment to affect the perception of object properties
in 2D images.

Size Illusions on the Open Prairie

Begin with an image that has zero-point perspective. I've selected an image of the North
Dakota prairie in Figure 7.7, but any image like this that depicts just a flat ground plane

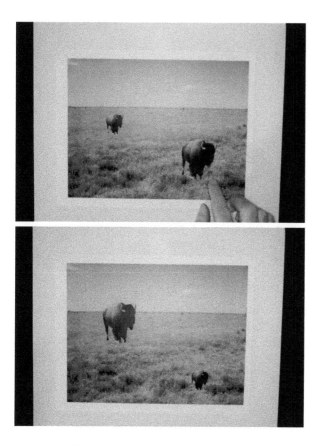

Figure 7.7 The horizon line in this image combined with the texture gradient of the prairie grass provide strong enough monocular cues that height in the image plane ends up used as a proxy for depth. This can lead to strange size inferences for objects of objectively different sizes places at varying heights in the picture. Photo by the author.

and the sky will do. In my case, starting with the image of a flat, grassy prairie you can see that I've cut out some bison (pronounced with a "z" in the middle if you want to sound like you're from North Dakota) of various sizes as well. Whatever kind of zero-point perspective image you have chosen, find an object like this that you can scale up or down to two different sizes, and cut it out so you can slide it around on your scene photograph.

A zero-point perspective image lacks a single vanishing point, but nonetheless may have texture cues (larger elements towards the bottom of the page and smaller elements as we move upwards) that indicate a receding ground place under an open sky and a horizon line that tells you where the sky meets the Earth. These two-dimensional features provide some evidence for your visual system to make some guesses about how position in the image plane relates to depth. To see an interesting consequence of this inferential process, we'll place our cut-out objects of different sizes in some different parts of the scene to see how they look to us with regard to their size.

In my case, I've placed my two bison in Figure 7.7 in different positions relative to the horizon line to see how their relative size appears to change as I move them around. You should find that while a large bison near the bottom accompanied by a small bison closer to the horizon line makes them look similar in size (see top image in Figure 7.7), switching those positions leads to the appearance of both a gigantic and a microscopic animal. Try moving your own shapes around on the page to confirm that the key issue here is how close each object is to the horizon line (which serves as a collection of vanishing points) rather than the horizontal position of the bison on the page.

Changing the Size of the Sun with One-Point Perspective

To further explore how linear perspective cues and vanishing points in 2D images affect perceived depth, we'll try playing some of the same tricks with an image that has one-point perspective. In Figure 7.8 you can see that I've selected an image of some railroad tracks, with a set of equally sized red suns as our next set of stimuli. Again, you can use whatever kind of image and objects that you like, so long as you have a single vanishing point to work with in the scene and cut-out objects of the same size that you can move around on the page.

In my example image, we have a clear central vanishing point that the railroad lines clearly converge to, and we can use it to play much the same game as we did on the grassland: Place the sun near the vanishing point vs. far away from it, and you should find that it's apparent size changes a bit as you move it around. Again, the depth estimates affect where you think the discs are in terms of their distance from you, leading you to interpret their actual sizes differently based on their image sizes. Compared to my image of the prairie, in this case the horizontal and vertical position of the cut-out objects on the page should matter. The key factor determining perceived depth in these images is how close you are to the single vanishing point, which in this case is right at the center of the page rather than an extended structure like the horizon line in the prairie images.

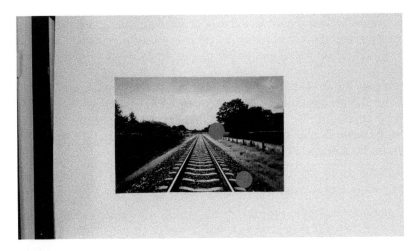

Figure 7.8 An image with a single vanishing point leads to the same phenomenon as in Figure 7.7, but in this case it is proximity to the vanishing point rather than height in the image plane that matters. Photo by the author.

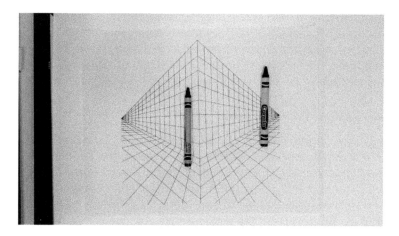

Figure 7.9 Two-point perspective offers the same potential for size illusions as one-point perspective. Photo by the author.

Rolling Some Crayons Around in Two-Point Perspective

The final image we'll use to examine vanishing points and linear perspective as they contribute to depth perception is a picture with two vanishing points. Once you've found a useful image with two vanishing points, I recommend finding two crayons that are the same length to place onto the diagram as shown. Much like our demonstrations with the prairie and the railroad tracks, proximity to the vanishing points serves as a cue to depth, with the crayon closest to a vanishing point seeming further away from you and larger as a result (Figure 7.9).

In all three cases, the geometry of linear perspective is being used as the basis for interpreting the layout of these scenes based on 2D features, leading you to further decisions about the position and size of objects occupying these spaces. These monocular depth cues are clearly quite powerful and can override other sources of information about object appearance. Critically, however, the use of linear perspective and other monocular depth cues like object size, object blur, or *aerial perspective* (the tendency for things that are further away to look more bluish in color) rests on specific assumptions about lawful relationships between 2D appearance and 3D layout. Those assumptions can be violated in many different ways, which means our subsequent estimates of depth can be wrong. This doesn't mean that our visual system doesn't work, but it does highlight how our vision relies on relationships between the environment and images of the environment that are true most of the time, but need not be honored in all settings.

What Is the Range of Binocular Vergence?

Besides using monocular information to estimate depth, we can also make use of the fact that we have two eyes that each get their own view of the world. In these exercises, we'll explore how the different images each retina gets of the same scene leads to a means of estimating depth. First, we'll test the limits of a somewhat cruder mechanism for estimating depth: The *vergence* of your two eyes when fixating an object at different depths. This is one simple way we could try to use the existence of our two eyes as a means of making guesses about the depth of the objects we are looking at.

Things you will need:

• Three people.
• A fixation object (a pencil or something similar will do).
• A tape measure.

Observing Vergence at Close Range

Begin by holding the pencil with the eraser end up in front of your observer's eyes at a distance of about 12" or so. Ask them to look directly at the eraser. Once they have done so, slowly move the pencil closer to their face until it is about 6"–8" away, then slowly move it back to the original position and further away until it is about 18" away from them. You should be able to see their eyes cross as the object approaches their face and then drift apart as the pencil moves further away (Figure 7.10).

The angle that the two eyes each make to turn towards the fixated object is the *vergence angle*. This is a potentially useful cue to the depth of objects in a scene that doesn't depend much on what objects look like in terms of a 2D image, but instead relies on a physiological cue that provides an estimate of depth. If we can measure this vergence angle precisely, either by looking at the pupils of the two eyes or by making some measurement of the muscle activity that turns your eyes inward, we could make a very good guess about the distance between our eyes and an object if we just use a little trigonometry. At the very least, we could decide that more turning inwards means a closer object and less turning inwards means something that is further away. The question is, how well does this actually work over a range of distances?

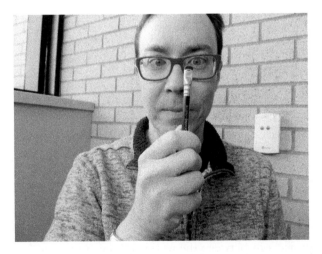

Figure 7.10 Vergence movements lead to a cross-eyed appearance as fixated objects approach the observer. Photo by the author.

Testing the Range of Vergence Cues to Depth

Here is where your team of three people comes into play. We've already seen that the eyes cross and diverge as objects move closer or further toward an observer. Eventually, however, the eyes must get far enough apart that it's tough to see any further change in their vergence angle. To estimate this, start with one person holding the pencil at the initial 12" distance from one team member's face and the third team member watching the observer's eyes. Move the pencil closer to confirm that the spotter can see the convergence of the eyes, then slowly move it backward until the spotter can no longer see the eyes moving. Measure how far away you are when this happens with the tape measure. If you'd like to try and be more careful about your assessment of eye vergence, you might even try taking photographs of your observers' eyes as they look at the object at different distances. So long as you're careful to take consistent pictures, you may be able to determine how the position of the pupils changes and ultimately plateaus as the distance between the observer and the object they're fixating increases. You'll want to do a few rounds of this to confirm your distance estimate, and it's also worth moving the pencil closer in and reversing back slowly a few times around the estimated distance to confirm when the spotter can and can't see movement. Try it with each of your team members as well just for the sake of consistency and removing any idiosyncrasies in reporting eye movements.

My guess is that you probably found that vergence stops telling you anything new about depth pretty quickly, maybe even failing after just about three feet or so. This means that even though this would be a lovely geometric means of estimating depth, it can only help us out within a limited range. The information from the two eyes is thus useful for depth perception, but binocular cues also have a specific scope beyond which they don't work.

Still, understanding vergence eye movements matters a great deal for examining another cue to depth in 2D images that depends on using the information from the two retinae – a cue called *binocular disparity*. To elaborate on what this cue is, let's start by drawing a diagram of what happened with our observers' two eyes as they fixated on an object at some distance from them: Their two eyes turned inward by some amount so that the object they were looking at would be right in the middle of each retina. We can draw what this looks like from a top-down view in the diagram in Figure 7.11.

We've already talked about measuring the angle that the two eyes make as they turn inward. What we'll do next is think about what's happening on each of the two retinae given that the eyes are turned inward to fixate on this particular object. To be specific, let's imagine that there are two more objects in our 3D scene – one that is further away from the observer than the object they're fixating and another that is closer to them than the fixated object. Let's call the fixated object **F**, and then we can refer to the other two objects as the **Near** and **Far** objects. If we think back to our work with the pinhole cameras earlier in the textbook, we saw in those exercises that light could only travel from the environment to the retina by passing through the pupil. In our pinhole camera, this led directly to the inverted retinal images we could observe on our camera's viewing screen. In this case, we're going to use this same rule to determine where the **Near** and **Far** objects end up in both the left and right retina if the two eyes are turned inward to fixate **F** and light from all of the objects must pass through the pupils of each retina.

If we add lines for each of these projections between the world and the eye to our diagram, we see something that is interesting and useful. While **F** always ends up right in the

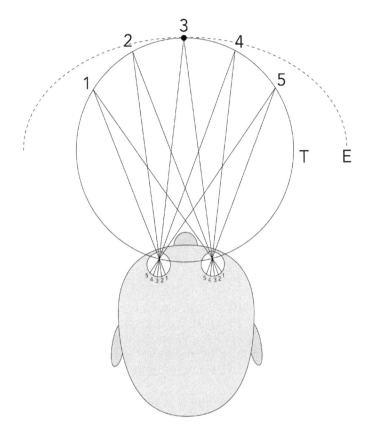

Figure 7.11 This curve, known as the horopter, is defined as the locus of points in the environment that will land on the same relative position in the left and right retina when we are fixating at the point 3 in the middle of the diagram. If we consider a point that is not on this curve, than it will end up in different places on the two retinae. This difference in position is what we will refer to as binocular disparity. Image Credit: Rainer Zenz, CC BY-SA 3.0 <http://creativecommons.org/licenses/by-sa/3.0/>, via Wikimedia Commons

middle of the retina in the left and the right eye, the position of **Near** and **Far** is different! Our **Near** object is to the left of **F** in the left eye and to the right of **F** in the right eye. For our **Far** object, the opposite relationship is true: The **Far** object is to the right of **F** in the left eye, but it is to the left of **F** in the right eye. The different positions of these objects in the left and the right eye relative to the fovea is what we mean when we refer to *binocular disparity.*

Like our discussion of linear perspective, this is a lawful relationship that follows from considering how 3D scene layouts are projected onto 2D surfaces and as such is another tool we can use to estimate depth from the retinal images. Specifically, if different positions in depth lead to different binocular disparities across the two retinae, then our visual system can try to work backwards from the images on the two retinae: Different binocular disparity must mean different positions in depth!

In our next exercise, we'll explore how this cue works by making some 3D images using anaglyphs. These are a tool for presenting your two eyes with different versions of the same scene, making it possible to control both the binocular disparities in two different images and the subsequent estimates of 3D depth that result from them.

Make Your Own Red/Green Anaglyphs

As we described above, binocular stereopsis, or estimating depth using the different images provided by your two eyes, takes advantage of some useful features of the projective geometry of image formation across two eyes. Briefly, objects and surfaces will end up projecting to different parts of the two retinae depending on whether they are closer to you or further from you than the point you are fixating at. Anaglyph 3D glasses work by allowing each eye to see a different copy of the same scene that contains the same contours, shapes, and textures shifted relative to one another according to the depth estimates we want you to make from viewing the images. The result is a 3D experience of a 2D scene. Here, we'll explore this relationship by drawing some anaglyph images ourselves (Figure 7.12).

Things you will need:

- Red/Green or Red/Cyan 3-D glasses.
- Red/Green or Red/Cyan crayons – This is a little tough. You're trying to find a good match to the filters in your 3D glasses, and I've yet to find a perfect option. For my money, most Crayola crayons that are Red or Red-Orange work for the red filter. For green filters, Crayola's yellow-green (but not their green-yellow!) works ok. For cyan, their Robin's Egg Blue and Sky Blue are also ok. You can get Sky Blue and Yellow-Green in the Crayola 24-count box.
- A circular stencil (or any other shapes you like) – the goal is to be able to draw the same shape consistently, so stencils are a good way to achieve this. You can still get good results by just drawing carefully, though, or using objects like coins as ad-hoc templates for drawing.

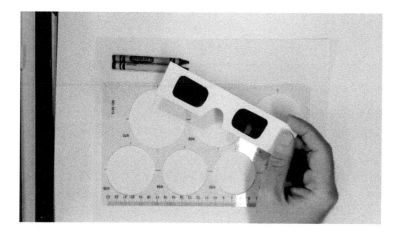

Figure 7.12 We can make red/green stereo images by drawing images with binocular disparity enforced by color crayons and matched viewing filters. Photo by the author.

Building Varying Disparity into a Simple Image

Our goal in this exercise is to control the binocular disparity we build into some simple images and then present two versions of the same scene to the two eyes so that those disparities are in the two retinal images, leading our visual system to infer depth from the 2D picture we've drawn. Our tool for achieving this critical second step is anaglyph 3D glasses that have red and green translucent filters over the two eyes. These filters allow us to use color as a means of controlling what each eye is able to see in the images that we draw.

Begin by confirming that the red filter of your glasses only permits you to see marks you make on white paper with your green/blue crayon and that the green filter only permits you to see marks you make with your red crayon. A simple way to check this is by scribbling with each color on white paper and then closing or covering one eye to see how well you can see set of marks through the red filter and then through the green filter. Chances are that one set of marks will look very dark to one eye, but the other set of marks will look very dark to the other eye. You may see at least a faint copy of the weaker marks, but this shouldn't greatly affect our results (Figure 7.13).

Now that we're confident our right eye can only see one of our crayons and the left eye can only see the other, we can draw a picture with binocular disparity manipulated via color. Draw some pairs of circles or other shapes in both red and green that are shifted apart from one another horizontally by different amounts. Make sure to put the green circle on the left sometimes and the red circle on the left for different pairs. Vary how big the gap is between the two circles as well, and fill the paper up with lots of different pairs of shapes. Be very careful to match the size of your paired shapes and to make sure they aren't shifted vertically relative to one another! If it's helpful, you may consider using graph paper to help keep your shapes lined up vertically so the only differences in position across your left and right eye will be horizontal shifts.

Relating Disparity to Perceived Depth

Now put your anaglyph glasses on with both eyes open and see what this array of shapes looks like. You ought to see some of the circles appearing to float above the page, with

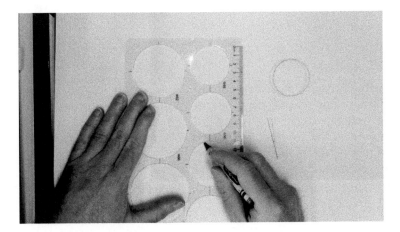

Figure 7.13 Draw matched shapes that are separated by varying horizontal distances. Photo by the author.

others looking a little sunken into the page instead. Again, there may be some double-image noise to contend with, but the darkest circle you see for each pair is what to pay attention to.

Once you have a pretty good sense of the depth percept, flip your glasses around to see how things change. You should see that any circles that were floating off of the page now look sunken in and vice-versa. Also, pay attention to how sunken or floaty the circles look relative to how much of a gap you included between the two circles. Specifically, measure how far apart your paired shapes are horizontally and how much each shape appears to float closer to you or sink further away from you. You should find the floating vs. sinking depends on which color is to the left in your paired shapes, while the amount of floating vs. sinking depends on how big the separation is between members of the pair.

Besides simply being fun to draw and look at, this demonstration highlights how your visual system can reason backwards from binocular disparity to achieve an estimate of 3D depth. This is a great example of your visual system taking advantage of limited 2D information to work towards an estimate of the richer conditions in the world that gave rise to 2D images.

Further Investigations

In the simple set of instructions above, we managed to make shapes that floated at different depth planes. There are more complex depth relationships we see in the real world, however, so probing the limits and capabilities of 3D anaglyph images is a good way to understand how 2D disparity information is related to depth percepts. Here are a few different things to try once you get the basic phenomenon to work. In no particular order:

1) What happens if you draw a red circle, but then put a green oval fully inside the circle?
2) How far apart do the circles have to get for the 3D percept to stop working?
3) How much vertical misalignment is too much for the depth to look good to you?
4) What does it look like if a shape is just red or just green? This should make it visible to just one eye, so what does your visual system decide this means for depth?
5) What if you draw a completely different red shape on top of given green shape (e.g. a green star on top of a red square)? What do you think this implies about how your visual system uses information from the two retinae?

DIY Stereo Photography

Anaglyph images like the ones that we made in the **Red/Green Anaglyph** exercise work well for conveying 3D relationships in a 2D image, but they're also limited in terms of how easy they are to make for complex scenes and limited in terms of the range of colors you can depict for obvious reasons. Here, we'll see how to make stereo images using ordinary photographs so you can take 3D pictures of anything you like. The underlying idea and geometry is all the same, but this technique is more flexible in a few ways. This exercise also helps to highlight how real images on the left and right retina support 3D depth perception (Figure 7.14).

Things you will need:

- A point-and-shoot camera – a phone will work just fine.
- A few objects you can arrange on a table at different distances from you.

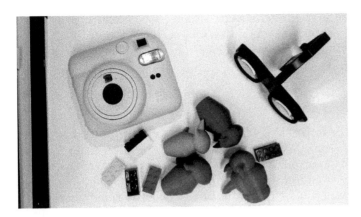

Figure 7.14 We can make stereoscopic images without colored filters by taking photographs that incorporate binocular disparity. Photo by the author.

- Access to PowerPoint or some other app that allows you to place images next to each other on the screen.
- A VR viewer – strictly optional, but many students cannot free-fuse! There are a number of inexpensive options available online, and these are also not hard to make with the right lenses and a cardboard box.

Make a 3D Scene with a Few Objects

We'll begin by arranging whatever 3D shapes we have at different depths in an interesting scene. I'd encourage you to use things that you can put on a table just in front of you, but they can be all different sizes and shapes otherwise. It's particularly fun to have some things with parts that stick out towards you or away from you in different directions.

These have a tendency to look a bit like indie album covers (see my art for the upcoming *With the Greebles* album in Figure 7.15) but, however you do this, it's likely to work well so long as there are things in lots of places.

Use Your Two Eyes to Take Images with the Appropriate Disparities.

Rather than draw images with varying binocular disparity for different objects, we're going to make stereo images that have naturalistic binocular disparity in them. To achieve this, we need to get ourselves two images of the same scene: One view of our scene the way it looks to the left eye and another view of the scene the way it looks to the right eye.

There are fancy and expensive ways to do this very precisely. You could build a stereo rig with two cameras, for example, set a fixed distance apart horizontally and gimbaled so you can turn them to fixate a particular object. We are not that fancy however, and we all have a limited budget, so we will instead use the following technique that works nearly as well: Choose something specific to look at in your 3D scene (I chose the blue Greeble figure in my images), and then hold your camera up over your left eye to take a picture of the scene. Next, hold your head as still as you can, keep looking at your target object, and move the camera over your right eye to take a second picture. This is a straightforward way to capture two images of the scene, each one with the unique view provided by one of your two eyes. Though it may not look much like it upon casual viewing, these two images depict your objects at slightly different horizontal positions, which is almost all we need to experience depth from these images with stereoscopic viewing. Go ahead and make some careful measurements in both pictures to confirm this. Objects that are closer to the camera and those that are further away should have different variations in left/right position in the first and second photograph.

Making a Stereo Image out of Your Photos

The last trick we need to play is to ensure that your left eye sees the left-eye image that you took and the right eye sees the other image. The easiest (sort of) way to do this is to free-fuse the images: Place the images side-by-side and either let your eyes cross to make them overlap in your field of view, or let your eyes drift apart to do the same. Note that this depends critically on how well you can cross your eyes on command, and/or how well you can allow your eyes to drift outward without focusing on something that is right in front of you. If you find it easier to cross your eyes on command, place the left-eye image on the right side of a page and the right-eye image on the left (as in the bottom images in Figure 7.15). In this arrangement, crossing your eyes until the two images overlap should yield a vivid sense of depth.

If it's easier to let your eyes drift apart, swap the left-right position of the images instead: Place the left-eye image on the left and the right-eye image on the right. Again, you're trying to get them to overlap with one another, but now we're achieving this by letting

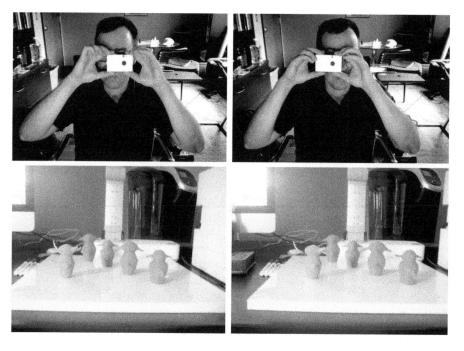

Figure 7.15 Arrange your objects at different depths and take a picture of them with your left eye and then your right eye. Photo by the author.

each eye look straight ahead at the image directly in front of it (turning your eyes inward here is *not* helpful!).

If neither approach works very well, copying the images to a phone or tablet and using a VR viewer to look at them should do the trick for you. Most VR viewers are designed for the left-eye image to go on the left and the right-eye image on the right, and the small lenses in these viewers help put the image in proper focus given the short distance between your eyes and the image. Hopefully one of these three options gives you a chance to experience the depth information in your two stereo images of your 3D scene.

This exercise highlights how readily our visual system uses 2D disparity to make guesses about 3D layout – even a crude pair of stereo images is enough to convey a strong sense of depth. The process still has limits however, which depend critically on how much binocular disparity ends up built into our two images as a function of the distance between our camera and the objects in our scene. To see what these limits are, you might try taking the same kind of stereoscopic images of your scene from different viewing distances to see when your ability to perceive depth between the objects weakens. Even so, an imperfect cue is still a useful one, and these exercises in drawing and photographing 3D images hopefully helped you understand how binocular disparity can be leveraged to yield meaningful estimates of depth.

Make Your Own Random-Dot Stereogram

I said earlier that our estimation of depth from the two 2D retinal images provided by our two eyes depended on some assumptions. In the case of binocular disparity, however, you may be wondering what those assumptions are. When we were talking about linear perspective, there were some specific relationships between 2D image features and 3D scene properties that we were assuming would hold in the images we were viewing. What kinds of relationships are we relying on when we use binocular disparity to achieve stereo vision?

A subtle assumption that underpins this phenomenon is that we are able to calculate binocular disparity in the first place. Specifically, we need to be able to match image elements (edges, textures, or objects) across the left retinal image and the right retinal image, or else we won't be able to decide what disparities are present in our two pictures. Though this may sound straightforward, the *correspondence problem*, as it is known, is complicated. Your visual system must contend with sources of measurement noise, similarity between candidate visual elements to be matched across the two retinal images, and many other confounding factors to yield estimates of binocular disparity.

Given the challenges in matching small scene elements across the two retinae, one approach to solving the correspondence problem is to forget about small pieces of visual structure and work with larger units of analysis instead. Specifically, how certain are we that binocular disparity depends on matching up small edges and little bits of texture across two complicated images? What if instead your visual system takes a first pass at recognizing some objects and surfaces in complex natural scenes so that you can match a dog, or a car, or a house, in the left retina to those same large objects in the right retina? Recognizing objects and textures before trying to estimate disparity might help us avoid some of the problems we encounter from trying to match lots of small pieces of visual structure across our two eyes.

This sounds like a neat idea, but it turns out not to be the strategy your visual system uses. Binocular disparity is an independent cue to depth that does not require recognizable objects to work. The random-dot stereogram, which you'll experiment with in this

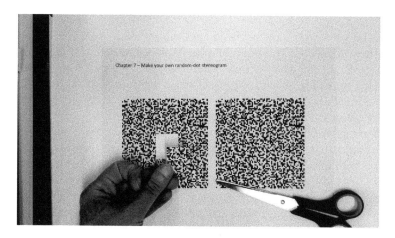

Figure 7.16 We can make "Magic Eye" stereograms with random noise images and some scissors. Cut out a small shape from one of your images. This will be the surface that we will have floating in depth. Photo by the author.

exercise, is a demonstration that pure disparity information alone – with no objects in sight! – is sufficient to elicit a 3D percept. This is the basis for autostereograms of the "Magic Eye" variety (Tyler & Clarke, 1990), which conceal a 3D shape or scene within a 2D wallpaper pattern with disparity relationships signaling depth information built into the textures making up the image. In this exercise, you will make a simple random-dot stereogram to show how you do not need recognizable or segmentable objects for your visual system to recover depth from stereo images (Figure 7.16).

Things you will need:

- Three copies of the same random-dot image (see the Supplementary Materials for an image you can use for this).
- Scissors.
- Cellophane tape.
- A VR viewer – again, strictly optional, but will help observers who have a hard time free-fusing.

Choosing a Proto-Object from Your Random Images

Begin by selecting a shape to cut out from one of your copies of the random-dot images. The simplest thing to do is to choose a square, mainly because it will be easy to keep this vertically aligned with regard to the second image in your stereo pair. My suggestion is to superimpose some guide lines (depicted in Figure 7.17 as red horizontal lines) onto copies of your random-dot images to help stop you from shifting your pattern around vertically. With these in place, even a complex shape can be cut out from the left copy of the image and shifted horizontally without adding too much vertical jitter.

Once you have cut out this patch from one of your random-dot images, confirm that you can find the same patch in the second image on the same page. That is, I want you to ensure that the same pattern of random-dots is present in both the left-hand and right-hand

Figure 7.17 Placing your cut-out shape on top of one of your images offset by some small horizontal distance should introduce the disparities we need to achieve a stereoscopic image. Photo by the author.

versions of the picture. This step may be a little tedious, but you should be able to identify some micropatterns that are enough to convince you that the patterns are identical and you've cut out a region that is present in the other picture. This matters a great deal because while we're not putting actual objects into this "scene," binocular disparity only works if it's possible to match patterns across the left and right eye.

Varying Disparity and Seeing in Stereo

Your next step is to vary the position of this image patch in one of the two intact random-dot images so that you now have a specific binocular disparity built into the two image. Again, the red lines are potentially useful here, but the key is to do two things with the patch you cut out: (1) Ensure that it is aligned vertically with where the same patch appears in the other image, (2) Vary the horizontal position of the patch relative to the horizontal position of the patch in the second image. For example, if you cut your shape out of the very center of the left-hand image, make sure you place it in the new image so that is either a bit to the right or a bit to the left of center. Once you have done that, I'd recommend securing it gently with a little bit of tape so that it doesnt slide around and then try to view these two images stereoscopically. As in our DIY stereo photography exercise, either crossing or diverging your eyes is a wonderful approach if you can do it, but a VR viewer will also work if you can't do either of these things. This is the rare case in which I'll also say that all this cutting and pasting is straightforward to achieve digitally with presentation software (PowerPoint, e.g.) and digital editing may help you use stereo viewers tailored for smart phones to help you see depth in the resulting image (Figure 7.17).

With regard to free-fusing, here is some advice: (1) I personally find that cross-fusing the two images is easiest. Cross your eyes until the two pictures overlap, then let your eyes relax in that new alignment. (2) Use the corners and sides of the random-dot squares to help you determine when you've achieved overlap between the left-eye and right-eye image, (3) Consider putting a small dot above each image, right in the middle, as an additional guide to determining the overlap. (4) Finally, if crossing your eyes doesn't work, you can also try wrapping cling film around your image to help you achieve divergent viewing. The key to using cling film in this manner is to look at your plastic-wrapped image with a bright enough light source that you see your own reflection in the plastic. By concentrating on your reflection rather than the image itself, your eyes should diverge enough that the stereo effect emerges. All of these take a little patience and a little practice, however, so don't get too discouraged if they don't work right away.

Regardless of how you get there, you should be able to see your image patch floating either above or below the page depending on how you positioned it relative to its starting location. Vary its position in the first image to see how the perceived depth varies, and you may try nudging it vertically or rotationally to see when your ability to see depth breaks down. The key observation here is that we have an image with nothing recognizable in it, and many, many small black and white pixels that could be matched to one another, yet your visual system is still able to match these patterns across the two retina and provide you with a 3D percept.

How does it do this? Though these kinds of stereograms have been called "Magic Eye" images, there is a non-magic answer to the question. Briefly, you may recall that we described cells in your primary visual cortex that were capable of responding when edges with particular orientation and size were visible within that cell's receptive field. That is, a particular cell producing a response was an indicator that an edge was present with an orientation and a size consistent with that cell's tuning to visual structure. That's a fairly crude summary of how your visual system uses cell responses at that stage of processing to make inferences about visual patterns, but it will do for our purposes. To understand how disparity can be measured without matching objects up, I can elaborate on the kinds of patterns cells like those respond to just a little bit. While some cells in the visual system produce responses to small elements like oriented edges by taking in information from just one eye, other cells receive information from both eyes and produce responses that depend on structures that are visible in the left eye *and* the right eye. Specifically, some cells in the visual system are tuned not just to the orientation and size of edges but also to the relative position of an edge in the left eye and the right eye. This means that the response produced by such a cell will depend not just on whether an edge in its receptive field is at a particular orientation or at a particular size but will also depend on whether or not that edge appears at a particular disparity across the left retina and the right retina. That tuning for retinal position in the left eye vs. the right eye allows cells in the visual system to produce responses that provide estimates of disparity from low-level measurements of oriented contrast.

There is, of course, a great deal more that we could do to describe exactly how this works, but for our purposes the key observation is that depth perception does not depend on object recognition in this instance. Instead, binocular disparity can be achieved with nonsense patterns, leading depth to emerge from otherwise uninterpretable 2D images. To me, this is an exceptionally powerful demonstration of how much work your visual system can do to look beyond the raw measurements of light to provide richer subjective percepts of the visual environment.

References

Ames, A. (1952). *The Ames demonstrations in perception* (pp. 1–130). Hafner Publishing Company.

Bruno, N., Dell'Anna, A., & Jacomuzzi, A. (2006). Ames's window in proprioception. *Perception*, *35*(1), 25–30. https://doi.org/10.1068/p5303

Gregory, R. L. (2009). Looking through the Ames window. *Perception*, *38*(12), 1739–1740. https://doi.org/10.1068/p3812ed

Pilewski, J. L., & Martin, B. A. (1991). Effects of monocular versus binocular viewing in the Ames distorted-room illusion. *Perceptual and Motor Skills*, *72*(1), 306. https://doi.org/10.2466/pms .1991.72.1.306

Tyler, C. W., & Clarke, M. B. (1990). The autostereogram. *Stereoscopic Displays and Applications, Proc. SPIE*, *1258*, 182–196.

8 Motion Perception

Like brightness, color, and depth, perceiving motion also requires our visual system to make an inference based on limited data: What does changing appearance over time imply about how things have moved in the environment? Though seeing motion may seem automatic, there is substantial ambiguity in the raw data supporting motion perception. This ambiguity can lead to systematic errors and biases in our estimates of visual motion that reflect key constraints on visual processing. To put it another way, perceiving motion is yet another inverse problem that is underconstrained, so our visual system has to use some heuristics to deliver a coherent subjective experience of movement. Throughout this chapter, we'll examine what some of these heuristics must be by examining simple motion illusions where what we see is not the same as what is physically happening. In the **Aperture Problem** lab, we investigate how limiting our field of view using a receptive field necessarily limits our ability to unambiguously estimate movement from changing appearance. Limited temporal windows for measuring changes in appearance yield similar complications, some of which we reveal in our **Temporal Aliasing** and **Flicker Fusion** exercises. Finally, we will close by examining the role of contrast in motion perception using a classic illusion called the **Stepping Feet Illusion**. In all of these exercises, the key insight is that, like other scene properties (brightness, color, and depth), motion is not so much measured, but estimated and inferred from measurements of visual structure that have important limitations in scope.

The Aperture Problem

Detecting and perceiving motion depends on deciding how the changing appearance of a pattern over time signals a change in position. The challenge in making such an inference is that this process involves a form of something called the *correspondence problem*: How do we match up visual features across two images? When we were thinking about stereo vision and binocular disparity in the previous chapter, we had to think about matching features across the left and right retinal images of the same scene. If we are thinking about motion perception, now we are matching visual features across images measured at different points in time rather than by the two eyes. Despite this key difference, this matching task is frequently underconstrained for similar reasons in both contexts. There are many valid ways to match up visual features that each indicate a different direction of motion. This is especially the case when we consider that the visual system measures visual features via cells with receptive fields that have a limited spatial extent. In this exercise, we will use small apertures to simulate the boundaries of a receptive field and see how the shape of

DOI: 10.4324/9781032691169-9

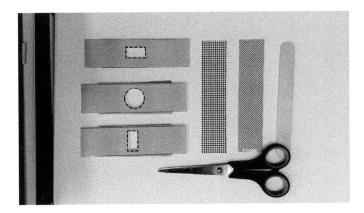

Figure 8.1 Paper apertures and patterns for observing the nature of the aperture problem. A small piece of wood or other stiff material is useful for moving the patterns. Photo by the author.

these openings affects the perception of a horizontally translating pattern viewed through the aperture (Figure 8.1).

Things you will need:

- Aperture and pattern cut-outs (see Supplementary Materials).
- Scissors.
- Craft popsicle stick (optional).
- Cello tape (optional).

Observing Horizontal Motion with an Unambiguous Pattern

Cut out the rectangular strips depicting different patterns and the different aperture cards. Fold down the flaps of the aperture cards after cutting out the shape in the dashed line. This should allow you to insert the patterned strips underneath each aperture and slide it back and forth horizontally without it sliding out. Taping the rectangular strip to a tongue depressor or other stiff material can make sliding the pattern a little easier.

Using the crinkled paper texture or a checkerboard pattern, confirm that sliding these patterns back and forth horizontally does in fact yield visible horizontal motion through the circular window. You can also confirm that the motion looks horizontal through the other apertures using the same patterns. So far, everything is fairly easy to explain: We moved a pattern horizontally out in the environment, and our visual experience of that event is horizontal motion. Though we have limited our field of view using these apertures, this doesn't appear to have grave consequences for how we estimate motion from these patterns.

However, we can observe a simple limitation of our visual motion perception with regard to time: Move the strip rapidly enough back and forth behind the circular aperture and your perception of motion should eventually give way to an overall impression of blur. This highlights the temporal limits of motion perception: Sufficiently quick movement in the environment can exceed the temporal acuity of your visual system, limiting your ability

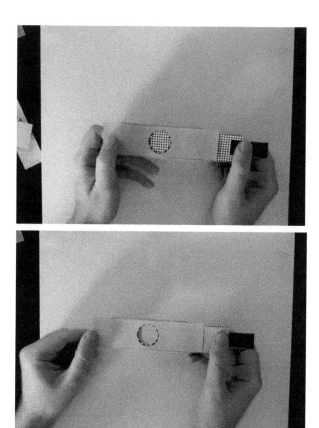

Figure 8.2 Moving the checkerboard pattern horizontally through the circular aperture should yield unambiguously horizontal perceived motion. Moving the oblique stripes horizontally will yield *diagonal* motion. Photo by the author.

to perceive motion. We'll explore this further when we examine **Flicker Fusion**, but it's worth pointing this out while we're here (Figure 8.2).

Illusory Diagonal Motion through the Circular Aperture

Now replace the checkerboard or crinkled paper pattern you just used with the pattern that depicts diagonal stripes (45-degree angle). Move this pattern horizontally behind the window and you should find that even though the pattern is really moving horizontally in the environment, the stripes as viewed through the window will look like they are moving diagonally. What's going on? Unlike our previous patterns, we're now perceiving motion that is at odds with what is really happening out in the world.

To understand why this happens, consider the data that your visual system has to work with as the basis for estimating motion. To keep things simple, let's imagine that your visual system gets to see one image of the stripes at a particular moment and will try to compare this to a second image of the stripes a short time later. Though the difference in the appearance of the stripes between the first and second point in time could have happened because the pattern moved horizontally, this isn't the only path the pattern could have taken during this interval to look the way that it does at each moment. As it turns out, movement in nearly *all* directions is a possible way to explain why the pattern looks different at different moments – the pattern could have moved horizontally, but it could also have shifted vertically, or at an angle somewhere in between horizontal and vertical. About the only thing that couldn't have happened is movement parallel to the tilted lines! This ambiguity is called "The aperture problem" in motion perception (Hildreth & Koch, 1987). Faced with this ambiguity, your visual system could either throw up its hands and say, "It's complicated," without yielding a subjective percept of motion. Instead, it makes an assumption so that it can settle on a particular motion direction: It chooses the motion that is perpendicular to the orientation of the stripes in your pattern. If you replace the 45-degree lines with the lines tilted at a shallower slope, you will see that the perceived motion changes according to this rule – the lines should move perpendicular to this shallower tilt. This turns out to be the slowest motion that spans the changes in appearance your visual system measures over time.

The Barber-Pole Illusion

Now replace the circular aperture with the rectangular openings (either horizontal or vertical is fine to start with). Again, move the tilted-line pattern horizontally back and forth and you should see something quite different than we did with the circular aperture. This pattern viewed through the vertical rectangle should look like vertical motion, but viewed through the horizontal rectangle the same pattern moving in the same direction in the environment should look like horizontal motion. This should also be the case with the shallower set of tilted lines, with very different speeds across the two rectangular windows in this case.

Again, what's going on? The same environmental motion yields very different perceived movement depending on which aperture we view it through. One account for why this is happening is that your visual system is still stuck with ambiguous data about motion (what changes in position out in the environment yielded these changes in appearance?) and has to use some sort of rule to dispel this ambiguity. Compared to the circular viewing window, these rectangles introduce an interesting imbalance to our changing pattern that the visual system tries to take advantage of to arrive at a new favored explanation of the changing patterns in terms of visual motion. Specifically, any aperture we might use to bound our view of these changing patterns provides at least some *unambiguous* features that we might try to use to estimate movement: The corners where the stripes meet the edge of the aperture! These corners can be (mostly) unambiguously matched across different views of the changing pattern, so if your visual system just pays attention to them, we might be able to get a unique estimate of how this pattern is really moving in the environment. This sounds great, but it also mustn't be a perfect solution to our correspondence problem – otherwise, we should see the true horizontal motion in all of these different scenarios.

The trouble is that in our rectangular windows, the different orientation of the window (a vertical vs. horizontal rectangle) leads to more unambiguous features along one side of the rectangle than the other. There are more horizontal corners when the rectangle is horizontal and more vertical ones when it is turned the other way. If you look carefully at the corners along each edge of the rectangles as the pattern moves horizontally, you'll notice that corners along the vertical edge slide vertically and corners along the horizontal edge move horizontally. What this means for your visual system's attempts to arrive at an

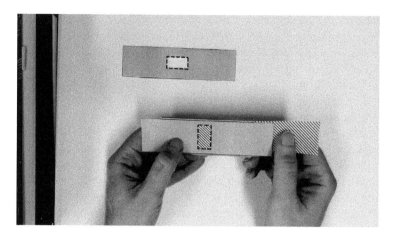

Figure 8.3 Varying the shape of the aperture will also change the perceived direction of motion even though you can only really slide the pattern horizontally. Photo by the author.

unambiguous motion estimate is that the length of each side of the rectangle is effectively a "vote" for the motion consistent with what those corners are doing. The horizontal edges carry the vote when the rectangle is oriented horizontally, but the vertical votes win when the rectangle is vertical, resulting in different perceived motions arising from the same environmental motion. Our original circular window has no such bias due to the rotationally symmetrical shape of the opening, so the motion depends on the orientation of the pattern alone (Figure 8.3).

What about Other Apertures and Other Biases?

Now that you know what's happening in these simple effects, try experimenting with different apertures. What biases are introduced by a triangle aperture, for example? What about holes with an elliptical shape or a fully asymmetric blobby shape? A particularly compelling type of illusory motion that depends critically on the aperture problem is the "Breathing Square Illusion" in which a rotating square spins behind a set of four squares arranged into a grid. This grid of occluding squares forms a plus-shaped opening through which the rotating square can be seen, and this leads to a vivid perception of pulsing movement – the rotating square appears to expand and contract – rather than rotation. This occurs for much the same reason as the phenomenon described above: The corners made at the places where the grid squares occlude the rotating square move upward and downward along the plus-shaped contours, leading to an overall estimate of movement that is either all heading outward or all heading inward. Other configurations can make the rotating square appear to be non-rigid such that it bends and deforms in odd ways as it moves (Shifrar & Pavel, 1991).

The key insight from these exercises is that perceiving even simple motions, like these involve estimation and guesswork, making motion perception subject to the constraints imposed by our tools for measuring changing visual patterns. Specifically, the aperture problem in motion perception highlights an interesting issue posed by the nature of the measurements made by the visual system: Receptive fields effectively break the image up into pieces, none of which in isolation typically offers enough information to uniquely recover scene properties we want to know about. Finding ways to combine information across these different local measurements or to take advantage of heuristics that support useful guesses about scene and object properties is deeply important to perceiving most aspects of visual experience.

Temporal Aliasing with a Spinning Top

In our previous exercise, we saw how measuring patterns over small spatial neighborhoods (apertures, which we used as a proxy for receptive fields) introduced ambiguity into the possible motions that could have led to the different appearances we obtained of some pattern over time. This ambiguity meant that our estimates of visual motion didn't always correspond to the true motion of patterns in the world. Here, we will see how measuring patterns over small temporal windows also introduces a type of ambiguity and also can lead perceived motion to differ from real motion (Figure 8.4).

Things you will need:

- A small top.
- A set of patterns to place on each top (see Supplementary Materials).
- A strobe light – easily findable at party supply stores.
- (NOTE – some observers may be made uncomfortable by strobe lights or be at risk for seizures when viewing them. As an alternative to the use of the strobe light described below, you can also view the spinning tops through a video camera to achieve most of the same effects. While it is a little less vivid than the stroboscopic stimulus, this may be a good means of including observers who are unable to work with a strobe.)

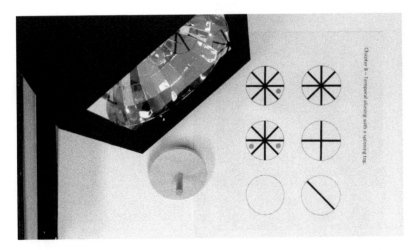

Figure 8.4 We can observe interesting temporal aliasing effects with a set of tops, some different radial patterns to attach to them, and a strobe light for sampling image appearance in time. Photo by the author.

Observing Stroboscopic Effects

Cut out the circular patterns on the next page and punch a small hole in the center of each one. It will also be useful if you can make small radial cuts in this hole along the spokes of the patterns. This will help you place the circular pattern over the stem of your top so that it doesn't fold or wrinkle. Begin by spinning your top on a table and observing what the motion looks like: At first, it should look too blurry to really see which way it is spinning, but, as it slows down, you should be able to see the clockwise or anti-clockwise rotation of the pattern. Like our first step in the previous exercise, so far, so good: There is a true direction of motion in the environment and so long as we don't exceed our visual system's temporal acuity, we get to see it veridically (Figure 8.5).

We will continue by simulating some temporal limits of neural processing by introducing a strobe light. This will allow us to clearly see the pattern on the top each time the light flashes, yielding a different estimate of appearance with each flash of the strobe. This manipulation turns our continuous stream of appearance data into something that is *sampled*, or represented by a smaller set of measurements. The question is, how does sampling affect the perceived motion of the top?

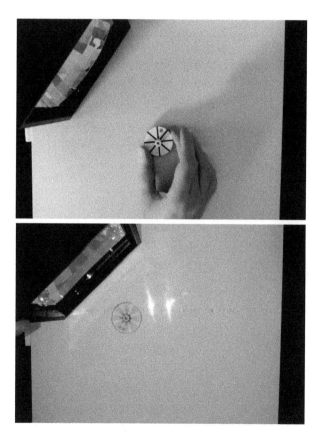

Figure 8.5 Set the top spinning and then observe the pattern on the top with different strobe speeds or letting the top slow to a stop. Photo by the author.

What you should be able to see is that by changing the rate of the flashing strobe light, the spinning top will not always look as though it is moving in the clockwise or anti-clockwise direction that is truly spinning in. Sometimes it may appear to freeze in place, or to reverse the direction in which it is spinning. This phenomenon is sometimes called "The Wagon-Wheel Effect" (Finlay et al., 1984) due to the presence of these aliasing effects in movies that depict spoked wheels turning (American Westerns tended to have a lot of these) – the frame rate of the movie imposes its own sampling rate, leading to the same effects that you should have been able to observe here. If you use patterns with a single dot among the spokes of the wheel, some strobe frequencies should be capable of yielding different motions for the dot and the spokes – the spokes may be frozen while the dot continues to spin, or the two patterns may move in opposite directions! Much like our situation with the aperture problem, we have a conundrum: How does the same motion in the environment yield so much variety in terms of our perception of that motion?

Again, we must consider how the correspondence problem is solved across different images collected at different points in time. The issue (again) is that there are multiple ways to imagine how these patterns could have changed over time to yield the patterns we saw with each flash of the strobe light. Faced with all of these possibilities, how should your visual system arrive at a unique estimate for your perceived motion? In the case of the aperture problem, we saw that your visual system used one simple rule to arrive at such a unique answer: Pick the slowest possible motion that accounts for the patterns we saw at different moments. As it turns out, this is the same heuristic that helps explain what we see in these exercises.

Depending on the relative speed of the top and the frequency of the strobe light, your visual system may be faced with a range of different *samples* of the top's appearance over time, each leading our "slowest possible speed" rule to arrive at different solutions for the motion of the pattern. For example, though the top is in fact spinning rapidly, we may get lucky enough to have our strobe light synchronized so closely with the top's rotation that the pattern turns a full 360 degrees between neighboring flashes of the light. What kind of motion should we infer from the two images of the top that we'd see under these circumstances? None at all! A complete rotation between two flashes of the strobe light gives us two identical images to consider, and the simplest way to account for that is to assume that there was no movement. This explains the freezing phenomenon we observed as the top spun. But what about backward spinning? To account for this, imagine that the top very nearly spins all the way around in the clockwise direction between two flashes of the strobe light, but doesn't quite make it through all 360 degrees. These two patterns will be nearly identical, but though they really occurred due to a fairly quick turn in the true direction, the slowest speed that accounts for the difference between them is a much smaller rotation in the wrong direction. Letting the slow speed win is what yields the experience of the top reversing its direction at some strobe frequencies (Figure 8.6).

As we saw with limited spatial measurements in the context of the aperture problem, limitations on how we make measurements over time also force our visual system to make some assumptions about the relationship between real-world movement and the appearance of those events over space and time. An interesting observation, however, is that the Wagon-Wheel effect can be observed in real-world settings in which there is no presumed sampling rate to consider! Merely watching rotating wheels on cars traveling with you on a busy road can lead to the same phenomenon (Andrews & Purves, 2005) despite the lack of any obvious sampling procedure like we have described. The presence of this effect in

True Rotation = nearly a full turn clockwise.

Perceived Rotation = a very small turn anti-clockwise!

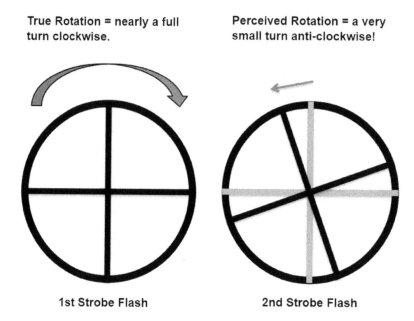

1st Strobe Flash   **2nd Strobe Flash**

Figure 8.6 A diagram of how aliasing occurs in the exercise described in this section. Because we only get data at sampled points in time, we make the simplest (slowest) guess about the motion that occurred in the interval between images. Diagram by the author.

continuous sunlight depends on intriguing aspects of visual processing beyond the scope of this book, including competition between motion processing units in the visual cortex that each signal slightly different things about the changes of visual structure over time. This is all to say that while some simple ideas about measurement and interpolation help account for some aspects of motion perception, there are other nuances to how dynamic visual information gives rise to subjective percepts of movement that we need to explain a wider set of experiences.

Visual Persistence and Flicker Fusion

The previous exercise about temporal aliasing depends on the idea that there is a limit to the temporal acuity you can apply to a dynamic event to record appearance over time. While it's not quite right to think of your visual system as sampling appearance in the discrete way that a strobe light does, your visual system does have temporal limits that we can measure via a phenomenon called flicker fusion. In this exercise you will use an apparatus called a thaumatrope to experience flicker fusion in two domains. This is a simple optical apparatus that has long been used to create simple illusory percepts that depend on the limits of your visual system's ability to resolve visual change across short time intervals (Jeffries, 1868).

Things you will need:

- Thaumatrope stimuli (I downloaded the pattern in Figure 8.7 from the US National Park Service, but you just need two pictures that will fit inside two circles of the same size).

- Cardboard (thicker is better).
- Scissors.
- A hole punch.
- Tape or glue.
- String.

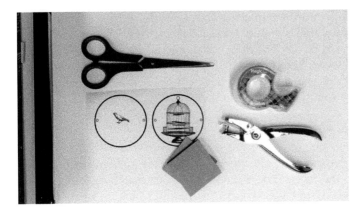

Figure 8.7 Cardboard squares, tape, scissors, and a hole punch to make our own thaumatrope device. Photo by the author.

Construct the Thaumatrope

Assemble your thaumatrope by cutting out the two circles depicting each of your objects and punching holes on the left and right sides so that you can thread string through each side. Tape or glue these images to opposite sides of a cardboard disc, making sure that one of the images is upside down. If you've done it right, you should be able to hold the disc in front of you looking at one upright image, then flip it over vertically to see the other image upright. Pull some string (or repurposed rubber bands) through each of the two sides to complete the thaumatrope.

Take the Thaumatrope for a Spin

Now that you've put the thaumatrope together, we'll investigate flicker fusion a little bit. What you're trying to do is spin the thaumatrope very quickly about its horizontal axis, giving your visual system a glimpse of the bird, then the cage, then the bird again (and so on) in rapid succession. You can either do this by twisting the string in your hands very quickly, or winding the thaumatrope up by holding the two ends of string and whipping the thaumatrope around in a circle until the two strings are thoroughly twisted up. Pulling on the twisted strings should lead to them untwisting quickly enough to see the bird inside the cage as the thaumatrope rotates.

This is too imprecise a device to test your perceptual limits very closely, but you can count the number of circles you use to wind the strings up, or the number of twists you put in the string before you set it moving. See if you can find a threshold of turns that makes the difference between seeing the unified image vs. the two separate sides unfused.

Flicker Fusion with Color

Besides superimposing different images, you can also use a thaumatrope to mix colors via flicker fusion. Repeat the construction steps using some red and green discs and whirl the thaumatrope around to see what happens when these colors alternate quickly enough. You should be able to see yellow resulting from the fusion of red and green via additive color mixing. Does the threshold for fusion here match the threshold for the bird and the birdcage?

In both cases (and others you can try by making your own discs), you're running up against the temporal limits of your ability to measure patterns over time. Visual persistence and flicker fusion are both related to the idea of sampling and acuity, but with regard to blurring over time rather than space. Your motion perception and the way your visual system uses data over time to inform spatial vision are both constrained by the resolution of your measurements considered over time, not just space.

The Stepping Feet Illusion

In our previous exercises we have considered motion perception in terms of matching features across images in time and space. The ambiguities in that matching lead to some specific heuristics that your visual system uses to estimate motion which we've observed in our previous exercises. There are other features of object and scene appearance that affect the perception of motion, however, and we will explore just one of those (contrast relationships) in this simple analog version of a classic illusion (Anstis, 2001).

Things you will need:

- A picture of vertical black and white stripes (see Supplementary Materials).
- A dark-blue rectangle and a light-yellow rectangle (see Supplementary Materials).
- A transparency sheet.
- Scissors and tape.

Making a Tabletop Stepping Feet Illusion

Cut out the small blue and yellow rectangles that you have and tape them to the transparency sheet so that they are parallel to one another, with one positioned near the top of the sheet and the other rectangle directly under it. To the extent that you can, try to stick these to the transparency using as little tape as possible so that only the rectangles themselves are visible.

Now, place the transparency sheet on top of the black and white stripes. A key observation to make here is that the contrast between the rectangles and the stripes depends on the position of the sheet. In particular, the blue rectangle is fairly low contrast when positioned on top of a black stripe, but high contrast when it is on top of a white stripe. By comparison, the yellow rectangle is high contrast when positioned over a black stripe and low contrast when positioned over a white stripe. If we slide the transparency horizontally over the stripes, we are also varying the contrast between each rectangle and the background in an alternating pattern: Whenever the blue rectangle's contrast is high, the yellow rectangle's contrast will be low and vice-versa. Try slowly sliding the transparency as described and watch the movement of the rectangles. Despite the fact that you must be moving them at the same speed, you should see the rectangles shuffle alternately like

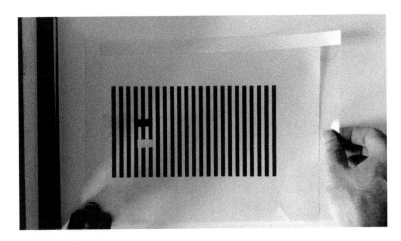

Figure 8.8 The necessary configuration for the analog Stepping Feet illusion. Photo by the author.

stepping feet. This effect will be hard to see if you are looking right at the rectangles and easier to see if they are in your visual periphery (Figure 8.8).

This demonstration shows us that motion intensity depends on contrast in a very direct way: Higher contrast corresponds to faster movement, while lower contrast corresponds to slower movement. This is somewhat different than the presumed matching across space and time that we explored in our other exercises and indicates an important link between the properties of spatial vision that we discussed in previous chapters (measuring light/dark patterns with cells in the LGN or V1) and the perception of motion. The varying strength of this illusory effect across the visual field also reinforces some of the ideas we introduced in those early chapters about the differences between central and peripheral vision, with peripheral vision being more sensitive to changes across time. Like the other properties of the visual world we have considered in previous chapters, motion perception thus depends on the original measurements our visual system was able to make of image change over time but also on how those measurements are used to make estimates about the world based on the image.

References

Andrews, T., & Purves, D. (2005). The wagon-wheel illusion in continuous light. *Trends in Cognitive Sciences, 9*(6), 261–263. https://doi.org/10.1016/j.tics.2005.04.004

Anstis, S. (2001). Footsteps and inchworms: Illusions show that contrast affects apparent speed. *Perception, 30*(7), 785–794. https://doi.org/10.1068/p3211

Finlay, D. J., Dodwell, P. C., & Caelli, T. M. (1984). The wagon-wheel effect. *Perception, 13*(3), 237–248.

Hildreth, E. C., & Koch, C. (1987). The analysis of visual motion: From computational theory to neuronal mechanisms. *Annual Review of Neuroscience, 10*, 477–533. https://doi.org/10.1146/annurev.ne.10.030187.002401

Jeffries, B. J. (1868). Remarks upon the principle of the thaumatrope. *Transactions of the American Ophthalmological Society, 1*(4–5), 98–101.

Shiffrar, M., & Pavel, M. (1991). Perception of rigid motion within and across apertures. *Journal of Experimental Psychology: Human Perception and Performance, 17,* 749–761.

9   Face Perception

We close our practical exploration of human visual perception with a brief look at high-level vision, by which I'm referring to tasks involving recognition and discrimination of objects, textures, and other nameable aspects of a visual scene. Among the broad class of visual recognition tasks that your visual system can solve, face perception seems to be unique in a number of ways. Besides apparently depending on its own network of dedicated cortical areas, the manner in which we recognize faces appears to differ from the way we recognize other things. We explore some of these special aspects of face recognition in the collection of exercises included here. In the **Squashed-Skull** exercise, we take a look at how well you estimate the configuration of a face by making some face patterns of your own. The well-known orientation specificity of face perception is put to the test by **Thatcherizing Yourself**, while our familiarity with the convex geometry of faces leads to the uncanny **Hollow-Mask Illusion**. Finally, we close with an absurdly funny demonstration of holistic face processing via the **Dynamic Composite Face Effect**. In this final chapter, we are lighter on theory than in previous sections, but hopefully you come to this section feeling equipped to use observations of new visual phenomena to guide your thinking about how your vision works. Remember that what you see is *data*, and you see a ton of interesting things all the time. With that in mind, have fun playing with some aspects of face recognition that set it apart from object recognition, and keep an eye out after you close this book for other exciting and puzzling things to see in the world around you.

The Squashed-Skull Effect and Face Configuration

The arrangement of facial features (the eyes, nose, and mouth) within the external contour of the head is one aspect of facial appearance that has been hypothesized to play a role in recognition. Both the first-order configuration of facial features into a standard face template and the second-order relationships between those features (the spacing between the two eyes, e.g.) have been proposed as geometric features observers might use to identify a pattern as a face and to label a face with an identity. Here, we will examine how well observers can recreate facial configuration, which is one way to determine the fidelity of these geometric features in visual memory (Figure 9.1).

Things you will need:

- The generic external face contour and face parts in the Supplementary Material.
- A picture of a highly familiar face (e.g. a celebrity or personally familiar person).
- Scissors.
- Cellophane tape or thumbtacks.

DOI: 10.4324/9781032691169-10

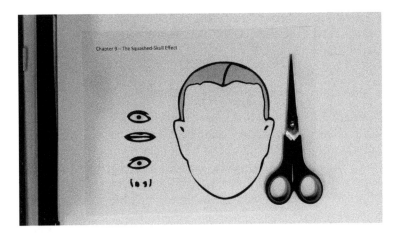

Figure 9.1 Scissors, clear tape, and a page depicting the external contour of a face and the eyes, nose, and mouth alongside. Photo by the author.

Build a Generic Face Portrait

Begin by cutting out the eyes, nose, and mouth from the first page provided after this exercise. Ask your observer to position these within the external contour provided so that the resulting face image looks like a typical or average face. Take as much time as you would like to construct a portrait of a typical face and when you are confident about the position of all of the facial features, either tape them down to the page or use thumbtacks to hold them in place (Figure 9.2).

Chances are that your portrait suffers from a common error in producing face images: the eyes and nose are likely too high within the outline, a phenomenon sometimes referred to as the Squashed-Skull effect (Edwards, 1999). The basis for this effect is still unclear,

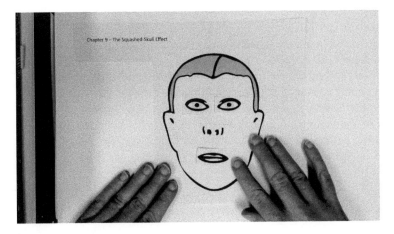

Figure 9.2 An example of how an observer might choose to position the parts of the face within the external contour. Photo by the author.

but artists generally learn specific rules for placing the eyes within a face outline to avoid this pitfall. Compare the portrait your observer made to a real face by measuring the position of the eyes relative to the top of the head on another person and comparing this to what was done in the portrait.

Build a Familiar Face Portrait

Continue by determining whether or not personal experience with a face affects the magnitude of the Squashed-Skull effect. Transform an image of a familiar face (either a celebrity or someone you or another observer actually know personally) in two-tone, using a graphics editing application. Digitally cut out the eyes, nose, and mouth and clean up the remainder of the face pattern so that only the external contour remains. Your goal is to make something like the cartoon outline pictured in Figure 9.1, but with a real face as the basis. Print out all of these items at approximately actual size, and repeat the face portrait exercise. In this case, you can compare the portrait to the original image to see how you or another observer did. While most people will still make fairly large errors in placing the features within the face outline to make a familiar face (Balas & Sinha, 2008) you will also probably find that it's not so hard to distinguish the real face from the portraits you or a partner make. This suggests that producing a face image is not quite as simple as adjusting your portrait until it looks correct to you: In this case, even though the real thing is evident when it's presented to you, it still tends to be hard to create a convincing image.

The Squashed-Skull effect (among other demonstrations) suggests that face configuration likely isn't encoded with enough fidelity to support recognition, making these geometric features not a particularly useful tool for face recognition. However, an intriguing feature of this effect is that while observers tend to make large errors when producing a face image, they tend to be much better at perceiving mistakes others have made. This distinction between face production and face perception is still not well understood and may be an important direction for future work in high-level vision.

Thatcherizing Yourself

One way in which face perception differs from object perception is that inverting face patterns (turning them upside down) tends to make them difficult to recognize, but doing the same thing to objects does not usually have as large an effect on recognition performance. The basis of this effect has been attributed to the holistic processing of face images, an inability to measure face configuration well in inverted images, or an inefficiency at measuring appearance in inverted images due to heavily biased experience in favor of upright face images. Regardless of the cause, the inversion effect is a consistent phenomenon in face recognition that, in the case of so-called Thatcherized faces (Thompson, 1980), can be used to hide absurdly conspicuous changes to facial appearance, as we'll see here.

Things you will need:

- A picture of your face printed to actual size (approximately).
- An Exacto knife.
- Cellophane tape.

Thatcherizing your face (or someone else's) is very easy: Use your Exacto knife to cut out the eyes and the mouth from the image. If you can, make these cuts so that the outline of each cut is as rotationally symmetric as possible (especially for left/right and up/down symmetry), and try not to cut through large features on the face like wrinkles or freckles. Once you have the eyes and mouth separated from the original face, turn them upside down and put them back into the face, or tape them over the original eyes and mouth in a new copy of the image. The resulting image will look grotesque, but turn the whole image upside down and it should look much less strange to you (see Figure 9.3 for the original in all of its glory).

With your Thatcherized face complete, show it to someone else in the upside-down orientation first, then rotate it to upright to see how the grotesqueness of the face becomes apparent only as the face nears upright. The relative inability to see these profound changes in appearance in the inverted face is a strong demonstration of just how much worse your face-processing abilities are when images are upside down. If you feel ambitious, try this with other faces that are smiling, frowning, etc. to see how Thatcherizing faces with different expressions may lead to a larger or smaller effect.

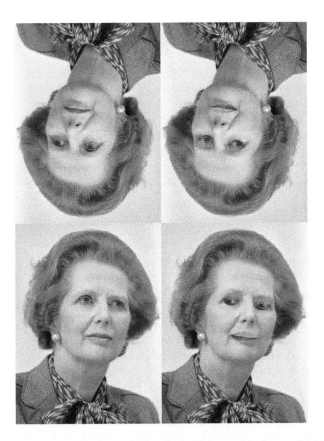

Figure 9.3 The original Thatcherized face, with former PM Margaret Thatcher's eyes and mouth inverted within the image in the right column. While the manipulation is highly grotesque in the upright face, it is much less conspicuous in the top row. Photography: Rob Bogaerts; Image manipulation: Phonebox, CC0 <https://creativecommons.org/publicdomain/zero/1.0/>, via Wikimedia Commons.

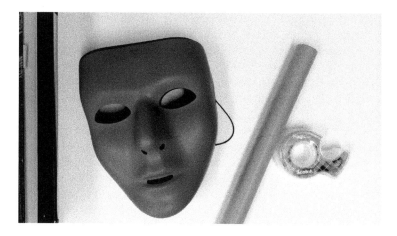

Figure 9.4 An inexpensive plastic mask like this one is ideal for achieving this effect. A cardboard baton or other sort of rod will be useful for rotating the mask in depth. Photo by the author.

The Hollow-Mask Illusion

One potential difference between faces and other kinds of objects may be the sheer amount of experience that we have looking at images of faces. This may lead to over-learning of the canonical orientation of the face at a particular spatial scale and biases in visual perception resulting from that experience. In this exercise, you will see how assumptions about the relationship between 2D facial appearance and 3D shape lead to disrupted motion perception via the Hollow-Mask illusion (Hill & Bruce, 1993) and probe factors that do and don't affect the strength of the illusory percept (Figure 9.4).

Things you will need:

• A plastic Halloween mask.
• A stick.
• Some means of attaching the mask to the stick.

The Basic Hollow-Mask Effect

Attach your mask to the stick or piece of cardboard that you're using to mount it, making sure that the face pattern will not be obscured either on the front or back of the mask. With that done, the actual effect is easy to obtain: With the mask facing you (or your observer) slowly rotate the mask around its vertical axis through an entire 360-degree turn. After 180 degrees, the mask will be concave with regard to the viewer, but you very likely will still see it as a convex shape with the nose sticking out towards you. This assumption of convexity will lead the tip of the nose and the rest of the face to be interpreted as turning in the opposite direction, an effect that will only be broken once the occluding edge of the mask blocks your view of the concave portion of the mask (Figure 9.5).

The pictures in Figure 9.5 don't really do the effect justice – you have to do this one yourself to see the illusory movement, but hopefully this gets across what you should be doing. Again, the idea is that your visual system assumes that the face is convex, leading

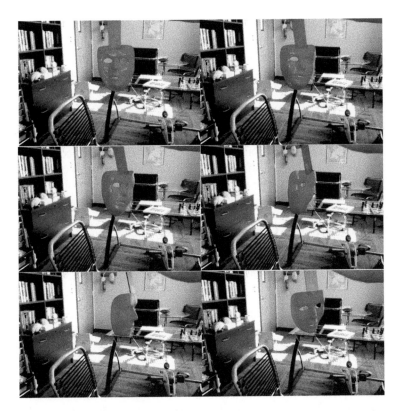

Figure 9.5 As the mask rotates slowly in depth, it's concave surface may appear to be convex to you. This misinterpretation of the depth relationships induces an illusory motion in the wrong direction. Photo by the author.

to an account of how the pattern must be moving that is different from reality. But how specific is this assumption of convexity to the face pattern?

The Inverted Hollow-Mask Illusion

Just what it sounds like: Try repeating the steps above but with the mask turned upside down on the stick. Do you see the same kind of illusory motion? People generally do, which suggests either that our inefficient processing of inverted faces is sufficient to support the convexity assumption or that this phenomenon is more general than we think. A way to examine that latter possibility is to see if you can get something like a bowl or other hollow, non-face surface to yield the same illusion. Try this out with some different shapes if you can to see what does and doesn't work.

The Specular Hollow-Mask Effect?

I'm including this idea just because I had the idea and had to try it, which is something I hope these various exercises encourage you to start doing. What if the mask has more complex texture, including more specularities that signal things about local surface orientation and slant? To put it more plainly, what if I smoosh aluminum foil onto my face to make a mask-like surface and try the illusion out with this stimulus? I was so pleased with this idea, but it totally doesn't work. Remember though, that these kinds of failures tell us about the scope of a particular kind of processing so what we've learned here is that the convexity assumption has limits that we've exceeded. If you feel similarly inclined, test other kinds of surface, face-like or not, to see when you do and don't observe the effect.

The Dynamic Composite Face Effect

One final key difference between face perception and object perception is that face perception appears to proceed in what we call a holistic fashion. This means that in several ways, observers appear to measure faces as one large pattern rather than making measurements of small parts of the face like the individual eyes, the nose, or the mouth. There are a number of ways to measure this property of face recognition in the lab, but this exercise is an adaptation of one of these paradigms (the Composite Face Effect) that is much more vivid and shows how small portions of a face image immediately contribute to the perception of a whole pattern.

Things you will need:

- An actual-size printout of a face – I recommend a serious-looking portrait done in oil, but go with what you like.
- Your face.
- A friend who is willing to laugh.

This one is so simple, but very effective. Cut the face printout roughly in half at the level of the tip of the nose (see Figure 9.6). I recommend cutting a small notch or dent at the nose so that the tip of your own nose fits comfortably into this space. Once you've done

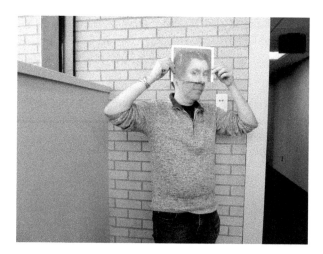

Figure 9.6 Begin by aligning the top half of your portrait with the bottom half of a real person's face. Note the small notch by the nose to improve fit. You will also want to pose so that your head points in the same direction as the head in the portrait. Photo by the author.

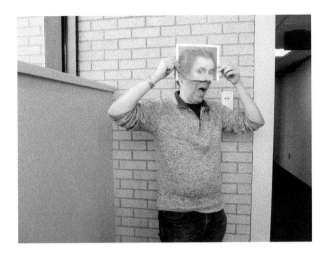

Figure 9.7 Moving your mouth should lead the eyes and eyebrows of the portrait to look different. Photo by the author.

this, hold the top half of this image over your own face, like a mask. Ask your partner to confirm that it lines up fairly well with your own face and head. A precise match between the top and bottom half isn't necessary for the effect to be measurable (Kurbel et al., 2021), but you may experience this demo more vividly by taking some time to line things up (Figure 9.6).

Now start making faces! Frown, pout, smile, and stick out your tongue. Though the top half of your head isn't changing at all, it will definitely look like it is as you make your mouth do lots of different expressions. In particular, the eyes will tend to look happier or grumpier, etc. as you make different emotional expressions (Figure 9.7).

The point here is that the changes to one part of your face seem to very quickly affect how the whole face looks. If your face perception was reliant on perceiving small parts, we might not expect such a rapid combination of visual information across different parts of the face. Instead, this strongly suggests that the face is perceived holistically with each part being used to make an estimate of the entire face pattern at once.

References

Balas, B. J., & Sinha, P. (2008). Portraits and perception: Configural information in creating and recognizing face images. *Spatial Vision, 21*(1–2), 119–135. https://doi.org/10.1163/156856807782753949

Edwards, B. (1999). *Drawing on the right side of the Brain*. Penguin Putnam.

Hill, H., & Bruce, V. (1993). Independent effects of lighting, orientation, and stereopsis on the hollow-face illusion. *Perception, 22*(8), 887–897. https://doi.org/10.1068/p220887

Kurbel, D., Meinhardt-Injac, B., Persike, M., & Meinhardt, G. (2021). The composite face effect is robust against perceptual misfit. *Attention, Perception & Psychophysics, 83*(6), 2599–2612. https://doi.org/10.3758/s13414-021-02279-0

Thompson, P. (1980). Margaret thatcher: A new illusion. *Perception, 9*(4), 483–484. https://doi.org/10.1068/p090483

Index

Note: Page locators in italics refer to figures.

absorption 5, *6*, 7, 15; blue light absorption 9; green light absorption 9; laser pointers 8, *8*; red light absorption *8*, 8–9; spectra 57, 58; spectrum, sunprint paper 35, *35*
acrylic lens 35
aerial perspective 112
Ames Window 103, 109; depth/motion confusion via 107–108, *108*
amodal completion 78, 84, 86
amplitude 7, 24
anomalous color vision 58
aperture *28*, *33*, 35, 36, 127, 130; *see also* circular aperture
aperture problem 126, 133; apertures and biases 130–131; Barber-Pole illusion 129–130, *130*; correspondence problem 126; diagonal motion through circular aperture 128–129; flicker fusion 128; horizontally translating pattern through 127, *127*; horizontal motion with unambiguous pattern 127–128, *128*; spatial measurements 133
artificial light 90, 91

backward spinning 133
Barber-Pole illusion 129–130, *130*
biases 98, 130, 142
biconvex lens 27, 35, 37
binocular depth 103
binocular disparity 103, 114, 115, *115*, 116, 119, 121, 123
binocular vergence 103, 112–113; binocular disparity 114, 115; far object 114, 115; near object 114, 115; vergence at close range 113, *113*; vergence range cues to depth 114–116
binocular vision 49
blind spot 47; binocular vision 49; "filling in" 48, 50, *50*; monocular vision 49; receptive field 48; retinal blind spot 45, 48–50, *50*; visual angle 49, *49*, 50
blood vessel 45–47
blue laser 8, 15, 53

blue laser pointer *10*, *13*, *51*, 54
blue light 5, 15, 21, 54
blue light absorption 9
blurry edge 100
"Breathing Square Illusion" 130
brightness 32, 90, 92–97, 99

center-surround structure 66, 68, 69, *70*, 71, 72
central vision 56, 65, 66, 69–70
central visual acuity 64
central *vs.* peripheral vision 61–64, *63*
chromatic center-surround responses 70
chromatic sensitivity 65–66
circular aperture 127, *128*; diagonal motion through 128–129
collimated light 40
collimated light source 40
color 5, 6, 58, 91, 92, 96, 99; change 91; gel 95, 97; illuminated by sunlight 23; of lights 7, 9, 10–13, 17, *20*, 21; metameric color 21; neon color spreading *see* neon color spreading; sensitivity 61, 65, 66
color-blindness 58
color constancy 91–92, 101; on black/white gradient 92–93; "Mondrian" image 98, *99*; "No Red Pixel Strawberries" 95, *95*, 97, *97*, 99; object knowledge on 97–99; simultaneous color contrast 93–94; spatial scale in 90, 91, 94–99
concave lens 38
cones 45, 56, 62, 66; absorption functions 57, *57*; absorption spectra 58; distribution 56, *56*; green cones 66; long-wavelength cone 58, 59, *59*, 67
constructive interference 19
contrast sensitivity function (CSF) 74, 75; contrast threshold for different spatial frequencies 75, *76*; light/dark contrast 76; measurement *75*, 75–76; primary visual cortex 76; testing 74–75; typical shape 76, *77*

convergence *47*, 62, *63*, 65, 67
convergence ratio 62
convex lens 38
convex prism 14
cornea 35, 36, 38–40
correcting myopia 26, 36
correspondence problem 121, 126, 133
crystalline lens 35, 36
CSF *see* contrast sensitivity function
curved lenses 14, *15*
curved surface 12
cyanotype 45, *51*

dark marker 100, 101, *101*
depth perception: Ames Window, depth/
    motion confusion via 107–108, *108*;
    binocular depth 103; binocular vergence
    see binocular vergence; disparity 117–118;
    DIY stereo photography 118–121, *119*,
    120; linear perspective *see* linear perspective;
    Model Ames Room 103–107, *104–106*;
    monocular depth 103, 112; random-dot
    stereogram 121–124; red/green anaglyphs
    116, *116*, 118
destructive interference 19, *19*
diagonal motion *128*; through circular aperture
    128–129
dichromatism 58
diffraction 6; for different colors 20–21,
    20; grating 17, 20, 21, 22, *22*, *23*; light
    waves bend 19–20, *19*; spectroscopy *see*
    spectroscopy; water waves bend 17–19, *18*
digital color picker 95, 96
digital display 2
digital resources 2
disparity 124; to perceived depth 117–118; into
    simple image 117; 3D anaglyph images 118;
    2D disparity information 118, 122; *see also*
    binocular disparity
diverging light 40
DIY stereo photography 123; image out of
    photos 120–121; images with disparities 119,
    120; red/green anaglyph 118; stereoscopic
    images 118, *119*; 3D scene with objects 119
downstream color processing 96
dynamic composite face effect 138, *144*,
    144–145, *145*

emission 5, *6*
entoptic phenomenon 45

face perception: dynamic composite face effect
    144, 144–145, *145*; familiar face portrait
    140; generic face portrait 139–141; hollow-
    mask illusion 142–144; Thatcherized faces
    140–141, *141*

familiar face portrait 140
"Fech Deck" 4
Ferwerda, James 4
"filling in" 48, 50, *50*
flicker fusion 126, 128, 134–136
floaters 45
focal length 14, *15*, 35, 38
fovea 62, 115
Frisby, John 3

generic face portrait 139–141
geniculostriate pathway 61
geometric optics 13, 26, 37
Gestalt principle 81, 83, 84
Gestalt psychologist 78, 83
Gestalt Telephone 79
grayscale grid 69
grayscale pattern 69, 70
green cones 66
green gel 97
green laser 53
green light 15, 54
green light absorption 9

Hermann grid 61, 68, *68*, 70–72
heuristics 78–81, 83, 89, 126, 131
hollow-mask illusion 138; hollow-mask effect
    142–143; inverted hollow-mask illusion 143;
    specular hollow-mask effect 143–144
horizontal orientation filtering 72–74
horopter curve 114, *115*

illusory contours and shapes: on complex
    backgrounds 86; illusory 3D volumes
    with 2D inducers 86–87, *87*; on uniform
    background 84–86
illusory volumes 78, 84–87, *87*
image formation, eye 2, 24, 26; inverted retinal
    image 39–43; iris 29; pinhole camera *see*
    pinhole camera; pinhole optics 27–36; pupil
    29, 29–30; retina *see* retina; sclera 29, 36, 38,
    39; in small camera obscura 26, *26*
image illumination 91, 99–102, *101*
image reflectance 99–102, *101*
incident angles 11
instant contrast sensitivity 61; testing 74–75;
    measurement 75–76
inverse problems 90, 102, 126
inversion effect 140
inverted hollow-mask illusion 143
inverted retinal image 26, 39–43, 114
iris 29

Kanizsa Pac-Men 84
Kanizsa triangle 84
Kitaoka, A. 95, *95*

Land, Edwin 98
Landolt C pattern 64, 65
laser pointers 8, *8*, 9, 13, 17, 19, 22, 51, 53
lateral geniculate nucleus (LGN) 61, *62*, *63*, 66–68, 70, 71, 74, 76
Law of Reflection *10*, 11–13, *12*, 16
LEDs 22–24, 30, 31
lenticular film 72, 73, *73*
LGN *see* lateral geniculate nucleus
light 5, 34, 48; absorption 5, *6*, 7–9; amplitude 24; bullet 6; emission 5, *6*; particle 6–7; reflection 5, *6*, 9–13, *10–12*; refraction 5, *6*, *13–15*, 13–17; spectrum 24; wave 7, 18, 19, *19*, 21; wavelength 24
light intensity 68; measurements 95; photopigment response vary with *52*, 52–53; spatial arrangement of 68
light wavelength: longer wavelength 21; photopigment response vary with 53–59; smaller wavelength 21, *55*, 55
light waves bend 18; through diffraction 19–20, *19*
linear perspective 107, 108–109, *109*; rolling crayons in two-point perspective 112; size illusions on open prairie 109–111, *110*; sun with one-point perspective, size changing *111*, 111–112; 3D images 109; 2D images 109
long-wavelength cone 58, 59, *59*

"Magic Eye" stereograms 122, *122*, 124
magnocellular layer 67–69
metameric color 21
metamerism 22
metamers 58
Metzger's Tiny Drawings 78, 81–84, *82*, *83*
Model Ames Room 103–105, *104*, *105*; build model room 105; objects in room 105–106, *106*; photographs 106–107; 3D appearance 107; 2D structure 107
"Mondrian" image 98, *99*
monochromatism 58
monocular depth 103, 106, 112
monocular vision 49
motion intensity 137
motion perception 130; aperture problem 126–131, *128*, *130*; flicker fusion 134–136; stepping feet illusion 126, 136–137, *137*; temporal aliasing *see* temporal aliasing; visual persistence 134–135
myopia 26, 36, 38

neon color spreading 87–88, *88*; color and contrast 88–89; elicit neon color spreading 88, *89*
"No Red Pixel Strawberries" 95, *95*, 97, *97*, 99

OFF-Center cell 69, *70*
ON-Center cell 69, *70*
orientation filtering 71–72; horizontal orientation filtering 72–74; lab 61; vertical orientation filtering 72–74
outer segment 56

Pac-Man elements *85*, 86
Pac-Man inducer 84
Pac-Man shapes 84, *85*
Palmer, L. A. 4
Palmer, S. E. 4
particle 6–7
parvocellular layers 67, 68
perceptual constancy 90, 91, 94, 96
perceptual organization 78, 83, 84
peripheral vision 65, 137; central *vs.* 61–64, *63*, 66; illusory dots in 69–70
peripheral visual acuity 64–65
periphery 56, 62, 65, 66, 137
photometer 94
photopigment response: vary with light intensity *52*, 52–53; vary with wavelength 53–59
photoreceptors 42, 44, 51, 57, 61, 62, 66, *67*, 64, 65, 90, 91
pinhole camera 26, 44; building *27*, 27–30, *28*; image quality improvement 32–36, *33*, *34*; myopia in 36–39; pringles pinhole camera *37*, 37–39; testing 30–32, *31*, *32*; two-hole pinhole camera 34
pinhole optics *see* pinhole camera
polarization 7
pragnanz 78, *80*, 81
Pragnanz Telephone 78, 79, 81; Gestalt Telephone 79; quick "calls" with set of observers 79–81
primary visual cortex 61, 72, 76, 84
pringles pinhole camera *37*, 37–39
pringles tube 36, *36*, 37
prism 34, *35*, 35; convex/concave prisms 14–17; triangular prism 13–14
pupil 27, *29*, 29–30, 32, 34, 36, 114

Rainbow Peephole 17, *17*, 20, *20*
random-dot stereogram: binocular disparity 121; correspondence problem 121; disparity and seeing in stereo 123–124; "Magic Eye" stereograms 122, *122*, 124; proto-object from random images 122–123, *123*
receptive field 48, 61, 68, 69
red filter 116, 117
red/green anaglyphs 116, *116*, 118
red laser 9, 53
red laser pointer 8, *8*, 53

red light 9, 21
red light absorption *8*, 8–9
reflection 5, *6*, 9; different for different colors
    10, *11*; Law of Reflection 11–13, *12*; light
    bounces off surface 9–10, *10*; path light
    quantification 10–12
refraction 5, *6*, 21, 34; different lights with
    convex/concave prisms 14–17, *15*; different
    lights with triangular prism *13*, 13–14, *14*;
    index *16*; optics of refraction 39
refractive indices 21
retina 30, 34, 38, 39, 42, 44, *44*, 62, *63*, 94;
    architecture 45; blind spot 48–50; center-
    surround structure 66, 69; with collimated
    light 40–41; draw your own retina 45;
    entoptic phenomenon 45; floaters 45;
    photoreceptors 42, 44, 51; retinal blind spot
    45, 48–50, *50*; retinal ganglion cells 61,
    62, 64–66; retinal vasculature 46–48, *47*;
    shadows on 45–46; shadow with collimated
    light 40–43; shining light on 46, *46*; sunprint
    photography *see* sunprint photography;
    transduction 44
retinal blind spot 45, 48–50, *50*
retinal ganglion cells 61, 62, 64–67
Retinex algorithm 98
rods 45, 62; absorption functions 57, *57*;
    distribution 56, *56*

sampling 131, 132
sclera 29, 36, 38, 39, 46
Seeing (Frisby and Stone) 3
seeing center-surround responses 61, 66–69;
    central vision, illusory dots in 69–70;
    chromatic center-surround responses 70;
    classical account of Hermann grid 70–72;
    peripheral vision, illusory dots in 69–70
Sensation and Perception (S&P) 1, 3, *3*
short-wavelength light 54–55, *55*
simple completion effects 89
simultaneous brightness 90–92, 101; on black/
    white gradient 92–93
simultaneous color contrast 93–94
Snell's Law 16, 21, 34, 37
spatial frequency 74, 75, *76*
spectroscopy 5; with diffraction grating and
    LED *22*, 21–25, *23*; light contents using
    diffraction 22
spectrum 24; absorption spectrum 55, *55*,
    56, 58; cyanotype spectrum 57, *57*; light
    spectrum 24, 53
specular hollow-mask effect 143–144
spike elements 86, *87*
squashed-skull effect 138, 139
squiggles 79–81, *82*

staircase method 64
stepping feet illusion 126, 136–137, *137*
Stone, James 3
stroboscopic effects 132–134
subjective contours 84, 86, *86*
sunprint photography 45, 51; absorption
    spectrum 55, *55*; cones *see* cones; laser
    pointer colors 53, *54*; outer segment 56;
    photopigment response 52, 53; rods 56,
    56; short-wavelength light 54, 55, *55*;
    wavelength selectivity 53, 56

tangent 12
Telephone *see* Pragnanz Telephone
Telephone game 79, 81, 83
temporal aliasing 126, 131, *131*; backward
    spinning 133; sampling 132; with spinning
    top 131, *131*; stroboscopic effects 131–134;
    "The Wagon-Wheel Effect" 133
temporal windows 131
testing central *vs.* peripheral vision 61–64
texture patterns 50
thalamus 61, 66
Thatcher, Margaret 141, *141*
Thatcherized faces 140, *141*
thaumatrope 134–136, *135*
"#TheDress" 98
"The Wagon-Wheel Effect" 133
3D volumes 86–87
threshold 64, 65, 85, 136
transduction 44, 51
2D inducers 86–87
two-hole pinhole camera 34
typical V1 cell 72, 74

unambiguous feature 129

vanishing point 107, 109, 111, 112
vergence 112, 114
vergence angle 113
vertical orientation filtering 72–74
vision science 1, 2, 4, 71; *see also individual
    entries*
Vision Science (Palmer & Palmer) 4
visual acuity 62, *63*; central visual acuity 64;
    peripheral visual acuity 64–65
visual angle 49, *49*, 50
visual cortex 61, *62*; *see also* primary visual
    cortex
visual information 72; dynamic visual
    information 134; fragmented encoding 78;
    perceptual organization 78
visual motion perception 127
visual persistence 134–135
visual processing 30, 42, 61, 66, 71, 72, 74, 78

visual system 3–5, 42, 47, 50, 51, 57, 66, 81, 98, 100, 129, 133, 138, 142; "filling in" mechanism 48; heuristics 81, 83; illumination and reflectance 92, 99; measures visual features 126; properties 22; resolves visual change 134; texture patterns 50; understanding of reflection and refraction 24; uses photoreceptor 51; uses 2D disparity 121
VR viewer 119, 121–123
V-shaped path 10

water waves, through diffraction 17–19, *18*
wave: amplitude 7; polarization 7; water waves 17–19, *18*; wavelength 7
wavelength 5, 7, 18, 24, 96; of light, *20*, 21, 22, 24, 90; photopigment response vary with 53–59; of wave 7
wavelength encoding 55, 58, 61
wavelength selectivity 45, 53, 54, 56

zero-point perspective image 110

Milton Keynes UK
Ingram Content Group UK Ltd.
UKHW011629220924
448658UK00021B/396

9 781032 691121